**Prevention.**
MAGAZINE'S

# THE
# SUGAR
## SOLUTION
### WALK YOURSELF
## SLIM

**4 weeks to a slimmer, trimmer you!**

Edited by Michele Stanten, Fitness Director, **Prevention** magazine

RODALE

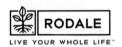

Every day our brands connect with and inspire millions of people to live a life of the mind, body, spirit — a whole life.

Chapter 1, "Easy As A-B-C Walking Plan," was created by Selene Yeager, a certified fitness instructor, author of *Perfectly Fit*, and contributing editor to *Prevention* magazine.

Chapter 2, "Eating to Energize and Slim Down," is a diet plan created by nutritionist Janis Jibrin, RD, author of *The Supermarket Diet* and a frequent contributor to *Prevention* magazine.

# Contents

Project Editor: Diane Gilroy
Editor: Susan Huxley
Assistant Editor: Katherine Riess
Editorial Assistant: Staci Foley
Cover Designer: Katie Seitzer

Book Designer: Maureen Logan
Photo Editor: Marc Sirinsky
Photographers: Hilmar (cover; pages 5, 8–10, 70); Mitch Mandel/Rodale Images (pages 31–33, 44); Kurt Wilson (page 7)

# Introduction

What do you love best about walking? Is it the thought that you are doing something wonderful for your body? Is it the way you feel as you power through your day? Is it because you suddenly look better and others are noticing too? Or is it simply the time you give to yourself each day, the way it reduces stress, clears your mind, and gives you peace in a way nothing else can?

There is no exercise more amazing than walking. You feel your body getting toned, stronger, and more energized with each step. You can do it anywhere, the costs are fairly low, and you see and feel the results almost from the first step you take.

Sure, sometimes it's hard to stay motivated. But don't let those little excuses sabotage you! In this book, I'll give you all the strategies you need to get started, maximize your benefits, avoid boredom, and slim down. I've even included a walking journal to help you track your progress.

Walking is the easiest, most natural way to strengthen and tone your muscles, your heart, and your lungs. Some say it also strengthens the mind, or at least clears away the things like stress that can get in the way of your weight loss success.

Think of this book as your first step. Now just keep taking one step after another, and soon you'll find you're racking up the miles, losing weight, and having fun—and nothing can stop you.

Michele Stanten
Fitness Director, *Prevention* Magazine

## CHAPTER 1

# easy as A-B-C walking plan

Looking for a friendly, straightforward way to get back in shape? We scoured the best research to put together the super-effective A-B-C Walking Plan. A-B-C stands for Accelerated, Body Shaping, and Cardio—three types of walking routines blended into one plan. You'll get intervals (to accelerate your results), circuit strength training (for body shaping), and tempo workouts (to improve your aerobic fitness and heart health). These moves also keep your metabolism revved so you burn more calories after you're done.

"If you always do the same walking workout, it may not keep you as fit as you'd like. You burn more calories and improve fitness faster when you surprise your body with a variety of workouts that include some higher intensity," says exercise physiologist Len Kravitz, PhD, of the University of New Mexico. A recent study of more than 15,000 men and women from the Fred Hutchinson Cancer Research Center in Seattle revealed that those who regularly walked fast or jogged were better able to keep off the pounds during middle age (when many of us gain) than those who stuck to the same slow pace.

The A-B-C plan rolls all these findings into one easy-to-follow program.

Each day—except on rest days—you'll do a specific A, B, or C workout. The basic plan will help you slim down, tone up, and walk faster without fatigue. And you can easily tailor the plan to meet your specific goals. *Prevention's* A-B-C Walking Plan has all the workouts you'll need to deliver the results that will keep you going for years to come.

# Three Workouts Rolled into One

## Accelerated

As the name implies, these workouts include bursts of accelerated speed. "High-intensity exercise will increase your 'afterburn'—the number of calories you continue to use up after you've stopped exercising. It also strengthens your heart so all activity feels easier," says Kravitz. The end result: You move more, burn more calories, and melt more fat.

Intervals can be as simple as speeding up between every other set of telephone poles or structured so that you need a heart rate monitor and a stopwatch. Fitness trainer and Walk Reebok training team member Leigh Crews prefers something in between. "I like 'ratio' intervals, where you simply walk hard for 1 minute, easy for 2, and so on," she says. "They're easy to follow and very effective." See "Intervals for A Workouts" on page 7: It includes options that range from moderate to intense. The goal is to push your body's limits at different speeds; this will help improve its ability to recover and do it again.

## keep the results coming

As you become comfortable with the program you choose (give yourself at least 2 weeks; you may need as much as a month), you can boost your results even further by ramping up your workouts as described below.

**A WORKOUTS:** Every other week, add one more interval to your A workouts until you are completing a total of five. If you are following the Walk Faster plan, you can get even more dramatic speed improvement by increasing the interval work and rest time in the A-Steady intervals. Increase the work portion 1 minute each week for 3 weeks; you should end up walking hard for 4 minutes and recovering for 8 minutes.

**B WORKOUTS:** Every other week, perform 1 more minute of one lower-body move and one upper-body move. After 6 weeks, you should be completing the entire circuit twice. Once you feel strong enough, try the more difficult moves for the Dip 'n' Curl and the Curb Lift-Off. Start slowly with these moves, and stop immediately if you feel any strain.

**C WORKOUTS:** Every other week, extend your C workouts by 5 minutes. Your goal is to reach 60 minutes. Don't have the time? Once you can keep a steady pace for 30 minutes, try doing the distance in less time. Aim to shave 2 to 3 minutes off your time every other week. When you can do the workout in 25 minutes, add more distance to get back up to 30 minutes.

# ■ Intervals for A Workouts

The A intervals explained below assume that you've been walking regularly for at least a few months. If you're a true beginner, your joints and ligaments need conditioning to handle the intensity, so do intervals only once a week for the first 6 to 8 weeks.

## A-INTENSE

Ratio: 1:4

Warm up for 5 to 10 minutes. Then increase your effort for 1 minute so your "work effort" is an 8 to 9+ on a scale of 1 to 10, with 10 being as hard as you can go. Ease your intensity to a 4 or 5 for 4 minutes of "active rest." Repeat for the number of times specified in each program. (See page 11.) Always end this workout with "active rest" or a 5- to 10-minute cool-down.

*"Because you have ample recovery time in this program, really push to keep the intensity high on the work effort," says Crews. It's also important to maintain proper walking form as you speed up.*

## A-BRISK

Ratio: 1:3

Warm up for 5 to 10 minutes. Then increase your speed for 1 minute so your work effort is an 8 to 9 on a scale of 1 to 10. Ease your intensity to a 5 or 6 for 3 minutes of "active rest." Repeat for the number of times specified in each program. (See page 11.) Cool down for 5 to 10 minutes at the end of the workout.

*You will have less "active rest" between work efforts in this workout, so each successive interval may feel harder, says Crews. If need be, lower the intensity of your recovery so you feel completely ready for your next work effort.*

## A-STEADY

Ratio: 1:2

Warm up for 5 to 10 minutes. Then increase your intensity for 1 minute so your work effort is a 7 to 8 on a scale of 1 to 10. Ease your intensity to a 5 for 2 minutes of "active rest." Repeat for the number of times specified in each program. (See page 11.) Cool down for 5 to 10 minutes at the end of the workout.

*This is a great interval program for beginners; although you have less rest, you're not pushing the intensity as high.*

*To make this more challenging, you can either increase your effort or extend the work portion to 90 seconds.*

# Body Shaping

These super-sculpting moves are designed to challenge fast-twitch muscle fibers that walking doesn't typically engage. Your muscles are made up of slow- and fast-twitch fibers, and regular walking works predominantly slow-twitch. You use fast-twitch fibers while strength training and during explosive movements like sprinting or jumping. "Fast-twitch muscles burn more calories and are the first to get out of shape from disuse," says Crews. "So if you have pencil calves or flabby thighs, these moves will shape them up fast." As a bonus, these exercises build strength and stability in your ankle, knee, and hip joints, so you'll be less susceptible to injury.

## TO GET STARTED

Walk for 10 to 15 minutes at an easy to moderate pace (5 to 6 on a scale of 1 to 10). Then perform the following 10-minute Body Shaping circuit. At the end of the circuit, walk again for 10 to 15 minutes.

## 10-MINUTE BODY SHAPING CIRCUIT

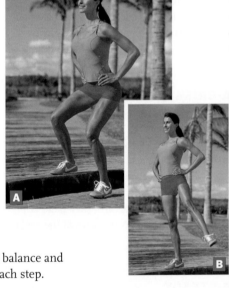

**CURB LIFT-OFF:** Find a curb or a small step. Stand sideways to the curb, with one foot on the curb and one foot down on street level. Keeping your chest lifted and abs taut for support, bend your knees and lower into a squat so that your legs are bent at 45 to 90 degrees (A). Be sure to keep your knees behind your toes. As you stand back up, raise and lower your leg that is on the street out to the side. (B). To make this exercise harder, add a jump: Squat as before, then quickly straighten legs and jump straight up. Land with your knees bent to absorb the impact. Repeat this process for 1 minute per leg.

Targets: Calves, glutes, and thighs. Improves balance and leg strength for a more powerful push-off with each step.

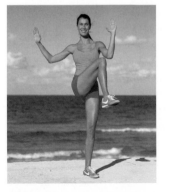

**STANDING CROSSOVER:** Stand with your feet a few inches apart. Bend your arms and hold them out to your sides, so that they form right angles with fingers pointing toward the sky, palms facing forward. Contract your abs, and draw your right knee and left elbow toward each other. Pause, and return to start. Alternate sides for 1 minute.

Targets: Quads and abs for a stronger core.

**BENCH PRESS:** Stand facing the back of a park bench or a low wall. Place your hands wider than shoulder-width apart on the bench, and walk back until your arms are extended and you're balancing on the balls of your feet. Position your feet wider than shoulder-width apart. Your body should form a straight line from your head to your heels. Bend your elbows, and lower chest toward the bench (A). Then push back up. When your arms are almost fully extended, raise your left arm straight out in front of you to complete the move (B). Pause for a second. Lower your left arm and repeat, this time raising your right arm. Repeat for 1 minute, alternating arms.

Targets: Chest, shoulders, triceps, and core for better torso tone and less upper-body fatigue.

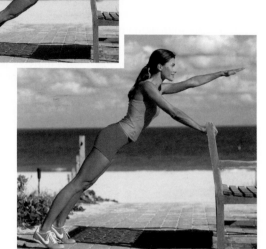

**WALKING LUNGES WITH KNEE LIFT:** On a level surface, stand with your feet hip-width apart. Keeping your chest lifted and abs taut, step forward with your right foot, and bend both knees to lower into lunge position (A). Keep your front knee in line with the ankle. Then straighten your knees and rise to standing, drawing your left leg forward; pause with your left knee lifted to hip level (B). Hold for a count of 3 before bringing the left foot all the way forward for the next lunge. Continue moving forward, with each step ending in a lunge, for 1 to 2 minutes.

Targets: Glutes and thighs. Also stretches hips for a stronger, smoother stride.

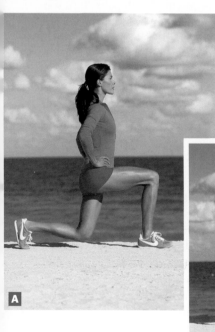

**DIP 'N' CURL:** Sit on the edge of a bench, and grasp it on either side of your hips. Inch your butt off the bench, and walk your feet out until your knees are bent 90 degrees. Extend your right leg with the heel on the ground and the foot flexed. Bend your elbows straight back, and lower your butt toward the ground while pulling your right knee toward your chest. Don't bend your elbows past 90 degrees. Return to the start. Repeat for 1 minute. Then switch legs. To make it easier, keep both feet on the ground while performing the dips.

Targets: Triceps, abs, and shoulders for core and upper-body strength.

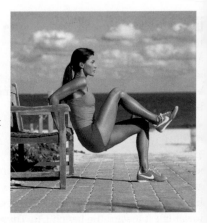

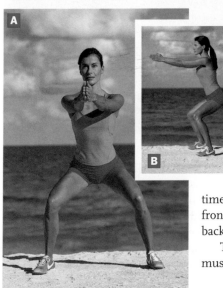

**PIVOT SQUATS:** Stand with your feet wider than shoulder-width apart, with your arms pointing straight ahead, palms together. Keeping your chest lifted and abs taut, bend your knees and lower into a squat, so your legs are bent 45 to 90 degrees, keeping knees behind toes (A). Pulse three times, lifting and lowering your hips just a few inches. On the fourth pulse, turn your body to the right by lifting the left foot and pivoting on the right foot (B). Pulse three times facing right, then pivot on your left foot back to front. Repeat, except this time turn to left, and then back to front. Perform for 1 to 2 minutes.

Targets: Glutes and thighs. Builds lower-body muscular endurance to tackle hills and maintain speed.

# Cardio

These walking workouts are the foundation of your program. "This is the solid, aerobic training that burns fat and calories and keeps you fit," says Crews. "The key is to maintain a pace that lies between somewhat hard and hard—about a 6 on a 1-to-10 scale with 10 as the hardest. You should feel like you can walk a fairly long time—30 or 45 minutes—at this pace."

The best part: As you continue doing the A and B workouts, your C walks will get faster—and burn more calories—but feel easier each time.

# Pick Your Program

With *Prevention*'s new walking plan, meeting any health goal is as easy as, you guessed it—A-B-C. Simply choose from the following plans.

## ◼ Overall Shape-Up

For the walker who wants to boost performance, shed a few stubborn pounds, and tighten up flabby trouble spots, the best plan is an even blend of A, B, and C workouts. After 2 to 3 weeks, ramp up your A, B, and C workouts evenly by following the advice in "Keep the Results Coming" on page 6. Or, once you're happy with your fitness and feeling comfortable, you may want to try another program.

### OVERALL SHAPE-UP WEEKLY PROGRAM

| Monday | Tuesday | Wednesday | Thursday | Friday | Saturday | Sunday |
|---|---|---|---|---|---|---|
| C 30 min | A-Steady* 3 intervals (20–30 min) | B 1 time through circuit (30–40 min) | Rest | A-Brisk* 3 intervals (20–30 min) | B 1 time through circuit (30–40 min) | C 40 min |

* Rotate through the three interval workouts, performing two different types each week.

## ◼ Beat the Blue-Jean Blues

A good walking workout burns fat and calories, but to really trim those stubborn lower-body trouble spots, you need more muscle-building B workouts. "Because you do these exercises during your walk, your muscles are already warm and ready to work. And you're energized from the sunshine and fresh air, so you may get even better results than you would by going to the gym," says Crews. After 2 to 3 weeks, ramp up your B workouts by following the advice in "Keep the Results Coming" on page 6.

### BEAT THE BLUE-JEAN BLUES WEEKLY PROGRAM

| Monday | Tuesday | Wednesday | Thursday | Friday | Saturday | Sunday |
|---|---|---|---|---|---|---|
| C 30–45 min | B 1 time through circuit (30–40 min) | C 30–45 min | Rest | B 1 time through circuit (30–40 min) | A-Steady* 3–5 intervals (20–25 min) | B 1 time through circuit (30–40 min) |

* Rotate through the three interval workouts, performing a different type each week.

# ■ Walk Faster

Keeping pace with your speedy friends is good for more than an ego boost. It also helps you burn more calories per walking bout, shrinks your waistline, and makes your heart and lungs stronger too. "A lot of walkers get stuck at a 3.7-MPH pace—or about 16- to 17-minute miles," says walking expert Mark Fenton, author of *The Complete Guide to Walking for Health, Weight Loss, and Fitness.* "By doing longer, fast intervals, you can break through that speed limit, hit 4 MPH, or 15-minute miles, and reach a new level of fitness." After 2 to 3 weeks, ramp up your A workouts by following the advice in "Keep the Results Coming" on page 6. Every fourth week, take a week off from intervals (sub in 30-minute C workouts instead). This break is an opportunity for your body to recover and rebuild your muscles.

## WALK FASTER WEEKLY PROGRAM

| Monday | Tuesday | Wednesday | Thursday | Friday | Saturday | Sunday |
|---|---|---|---|---|---|---|
| C 30–45 min | A-Intense 3 intervals (20–30 min) | B 1 time through circuit (30–40 min) | A-Brisk 3 intervals (20–30 min) | Rest | A-Steady 3 intervals (30 min) | C 30–45 min |

# ■ Build a Healthy Heart

Both A and C walking workouts are good for your heart, and combining them is even better, says *Prevention* advisor Wayne Westcott, PhD. "Research shows that prolonged aerobic exercise increases your heart chambers' capacity, and higher-intensity interval workouts make the muscle stronger so your heart can pump more blood with every beat," he says. Together they create a stronger, more efficient, and most important, healthier heart. If you're just starting out on a walking program, begin with 20-minute walks. Then tack on 2 to 3 minutes each week until you're walking for the prescribed amount of time. To make further fitness gains, ramp up your A and/or C workouts by following the advice in "Keep the Results Coming" on page 6.

## BUILD A HEALTHY HEART WEEKLY PROGRAM

| Monday | Tuesday | Wednesday | Thursday | Friday | Saturday | Sunday |
|---|---|---|---|---|---|---|
| Rest or C 20–30 min | A-Steady* 3 or 4 intervals (30 min) | C 30–40 min | A-Brisk* 3 or 4 intervals (30 min) | B (optional) 1 time through circuit (30 min) | C 30–45 min | C 30–45 min |

*Rotate through the three interval workouts, performing two different types each week.*

# Blast Fat

The three steps to weight loss are cardio, cardio, and cardio, says exercise physiologist Len Kravitz, PhD. "Every cell has fat-burning furnaces called mitochondria," he explains. As you increase fitness through continuous aerobic exercise, those mitochondria increase their function dramatically to more effectively burn fat." That means plenty of C workouts. After 3 to 4 weeks, start ramping up your C workouts by following the advice in "Keep the Results Coming" on page 6. After 2 months, consider adding time and intensity to your A workouts. Again, use the advice in "Keep the Results Coming" on page 6.

## BLAST FAT WEEKLY PROGRAM

| Monday | Tuesday | Wednesday | Thursday | Friday | Saturday | Sunday |
|--------|---------|-----------|----------|--------|----------|--------|
| A-Brisk 3 intervals (20–30 min) | A-Steady* 3 intervals (20–30 min) | C 30 min | Rest | B 1 time through circuit (30–40 min) | C 45–60 min | C 45–60 min |

*Rotate through the three interval workouts, performing two different types each week.*

**T I P**

*To increase your walking speed, bend your arms so your elbows form 90-degree angles, and then pump them forward and back at a faster pace than your usual walking motion. Don't let your arms swing to the sides like chicken wings or come higher than chest height. Take shorter, quicker strides, so your legs keep pace with your arms, and push off your toes at the end of each step as if you were trying to show someone behind you the sole of your shoe. Keep your shoulders down and back, your head up, and your abs taut.*

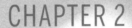

## CHAPTER 2

# eating to energize and slim down

**H**ow's this for a dream diet—a calorie count that will help you shed pounds and enough scrumptious, satisfying food to stave off hunger? In this chapter, you'll find a diet with six 1,600-calorie daily menus to enhance the slimming benefits of our three walking workouts presented in chapter 1 without sacrificing any nutritional needs. Plus, each meal plan delivers energy to burn during serious walking with a healthy balance of calories: 48% from carbs, 25% from protein, and 27% from fat (only 7% from saturated fat). Just pick the plan that corresponds to your workout for the day.

# Plan A

On Accelerated (A) days, you may need a little extra fuel because the speed bursts that are built into your walk increase calorie burn. University of Ottawa researchers found that women exercisers ate more calories on days when they did especially challenging workouts. So, if you feel hungrier than you do on B or C days, you have an optional 200 calories to play with, guilt free. Whether you use the extra calories depends on how much weight you want to lose and how much energy you have after pushing yourself.

You also get a sweet treat on A days. You could call it a reward for meeting the accelerated walking challenge, but there's a physical benefit, too: "Thirty minutes after an intense workout, your muscle cells are like little sponges, soaking up glucose and protein to build muscle fibers and store energy for the next workout," says Susan Kleiner, PhD, RD, author of *PowerFood*. "A sweet, milk-based treat, like a Frappuccino or milkshake, on days of high-intensity exercise will go to muscle, not fat, provided you stay within your daily calorie allowance."

## Day 1

### BREAKFAST
- 1 toasted whole wheat English muffin (such as Thomas' Hearty Grains) topped with 1½ Tbsp peanut or almond butter and 2 tsp honey or jam
- 1 c fat-free milk
- 1 c fresh or frozen unsweetened strawberries, raspberries, or blackberries

### LUNCH
- Smoked turkey and arugula sandwich (3 oz sliced smoked turkey breast with 1/3 to 1/2 c arugula and 1 Tbsp reduced-fat mayo on 2 slices whole grain bread)
- 1½ c crudités (red bell pepper, cauliflower, etc.)
- 1 orange

### AFTERNOON SNACK
- 3/4 c 1% cottage cheese with 1 sliced kiwifruit

### DINNER
- Spinach Omelet (2 omega-3–enriched eggs and 5 c [half a 10-oz bag] fresh spinach)
- Medium sweet potato or yam, baked or microwaved and cubed; optional topping: 3 Tbsp low-fat plain yogurt

**DAY 1 TOTAL**
Protein 95 g
Carbohydrates 210 g
Fat 48 g
Saturated Fat 13 g
Cholesterol 432 mg
Fiber 29 g
Sodium 2,148 mg

## SWEET TREAT

- 9½ oz bottled Frappuccino or milkshake (½ c reduced-fat ice cream with ½ c fat-free milk and 2 tsp Hershey's chocolate syrup)

**Optional Calorie Boost:** Add an additional 100 calories with 2 Tbsp nut butter at breakfast and a large (not medium) sweet potato at dinner. Add another 100 calories to the cottage cheese snack with a slice of whole grain bread plus 1 tsp trans-free margarine.

# ■ Day 2

### BREAKFAST
- 180-calorie serving of high-fiber cereal with at least 4 g of fiber per oz (such as 1¼ c Kashi GoLean)
- ½ banana
- 2 Tbsp walnuts
- 1 c fat-free milk

### MIDMORNING SNACK
- ¾ c (6 oz) low-fat plain yogurt with 1 tsp honey and ½ banana, sliced

### LUNCH
- Tofu and Watercress Wrap with Peanut Sauce (see recipe at right)
- 5 carrot sticks

### DINNER
- 5 oz ground turkey patty (broiled or sautéed) on whole wheat bun with lettuce, tomato slices, onion, and mustard to taste
- Chopped tomato tossed with 3 c mixed greens and olive or canola oil–based dressing (equivalent to 80 calories)

### SWEET TREAT
- 9½ oz bottled Frappuccino or milkshake (½ c reduced-fat ice cream with ½ c fat-free milk and 2 tsp Hershey's chocolate syrup)

**Optional Calorie Boost:** Add an additional 100 calories by having whole grain trans-free crackers (such as 5 Triscuits) with your yogurt snack. For another 100 calories, have 2 c sliced zucchini and a little minced garlic sautéed in 1½ tsp olive oil with dinner.

**DAY 2 TOTAL**
Protein 94 g
Carbohydrates 222 g
Fat 53 g
Saturated Fat 13 g
Cholesterol 88 mg
Fiber 33 g
Sodium 1,605 mg

# Tofu and Watercress Wrap with Peanut Sauce

### SAUCE

- 3 Tbsp natural peanut butter
- 1 Tbsp + 2 tsp fresh lime juice
- 2 tsp reduced-sodium soy sauce
- 2 tsp sugar
- 2 tsp water
- 1 tsp grated or finely chopped fresh ginger
- 1/4–1/2 tsp red-pepper flakes

### WRAPS

- 2 whole wheat tortillas (9"–10" in diameter, 180 calories each)
- 6 oz extra-firm tofu, drained, patted dry, and cut into 1/2" cubes
- 2 c watercress leaves
- 1 Tbsp chopped cilantro

1. To prepare sauce: Whisk ingredients in small bowl.
2. To prepare wraps: Heat tortillas per package directions. In small bowl, toss tofu cubes in 1 tablespoon of the peanut sauce. Spread 1 tortilla with half of remaining sauce. Layer with half of tofu cubes, watercress, and cilantro, and then roll. Repeat with second tortilla, and serve.

**MAKES 2 SERVINGS**

**Per serving:** 527 cal, 25 g pro, 44 g carb, 29.6 g fat, 5 g sat fat, 0 mg chol, 7 g fiber, 550 mg sodium

# Plan B

On Body Shaping (B) days, when you mix strength training with walking, you're in for another treat: a delicious whey shake. Consuming whey, one of the proteins found in milk, before or after strength training helps build muscle and increase strength, report researchers in Australia and Canada. In both studies, knee extensor strength—a good indicator of overall muscle power—was greater in people who drank a whey shake before or after exercising than in those whose shake didn't contain whey. Our special shake on B days gives your body a muscle-building edge with more calories from protein (30%) than other days. And, because both B meal plans also cut carbs and fat slightly, you stay within the day's calorie limit.

## ■ Day 1

### BREAKFAST
- 1 omega-3–enriched egg scrambled in 2 tsp olive oil or trans-free margarine on 1/2 whole grain bagel
- 1 c fat-free milk
- 1 orange

### LUNCH
- 1/2 whole grain bagel with 1 1/2 Tbsp peanut butter and 2 tsp jam
- 1 c fat-free milk
- 1 red bell pepper, sliced

### DINNER
- Horseradish-Encrusted Salmon (see recipe at right)
- 10 pieces of asparagus brushed with a mix of 1 tsp olive oil and lemon juice, pepper, and salt to taste, and broiled 5 minutes
- 1/2 c cooked whole wheat couscous

### POSTWORKOUT SNACK
- Strawberry Whey Shake (blend 1/2 c fat-free milk, 1 c frozen unsweetened strawberries, 2 Tbsp water, and 3 Tbsp vanilla whey powder until smooth, about 30 seconds)

**DAY 1 TOTAL**
Protein 117 g
Carbohydrates 186 g
Fat 45 g
Saturated Fat 10 g
Cholesterol 269 mg
Fiber 28 g
Sodium 1,037 mg

# Horseradish-Encrusted Salmon

**PREP TIME:** 5 MINUTES
**COOKING TIME:** 12 MINUTES

- 2 tsp + 1 Tbsp olive oil
- 2 salmon fillets (6 oz each), with skin
- 1/3 c dried bread crumbs
- 2 Tbsp grated fresh ginger
- 2 Tbsp bottled fresh horseradish root

1. Preheat oven to 350°F.
2. Brush ovenproof skillet or shallow baking dish with 1 teaspoon of the oil. Place salmon fillets in skillet, skin side down.
3. In food processor, combine bread crumbs, ginger, horseradish, and remaining oil, and pulse to make a thick paste. Divide mixture in half, and pat one half on top of each fillet.
4. Bake, uncovered, until salmon is opaque and flaky but not dry, about 12 minutes.

**MAKES 2 SERVINGS**

**Per serving:** 420 cal, 39 g pro, 16 g carb, 21 g fat, 3.7 g sat fat, 77 mg chol, 1 g fiber, 257 mg sodium

 **Day 2**

### BREAKFAST
- 180-calorie serving of high-fiber cereal with at least 4 g of fiber per oz (such as 1 1/4 c Kashi GoLean)
- 1 small apple or pear
- 2 Tbsp walnuts
- 1 c fat-free milk

### LUNCH
- Southwestern Chicken Salad with Crispy Tortilla Chips (see recipe on page 20)
- 100-calorie serving of dark chocolate (about 3/4 oz)

# Southwestern Chicken Salad with Crispy Tortilla Chips

**PREP TIME:** 14 MINUTES
**COOKING TIME:** 5 MINUTES

- 1 whole wheat tortilla (9"–10" diameter, 180 calories)
  Zest of 1 lime
- ½ tsp minced garlic
- ½ tsp cumin
- ⅛ tsp red-pepper flakes
- 1½ c cooked chicken, pulled from half a rotisserie chicken, skin discarded
- 1 Tbsp fresh lime juice
- 1 Tbsp olive oil
- 1 Tbsp (or more, to taste) chopped cilantro
- 8 c mixed greens
- 1 red bell pepper, sliced
- ¼ avocado, sliced

1. Preheat oven to 400°F.
2. Cut tortilla into quarters and each quarter into 2 wedges. Place on baking sheet, and bake until crisp, about 5 minutes. Remove from oven, and set aside.
3. Place lime zest, garlic, cumin, and red-pepper flakes in medium bowl, and stir. Add chicken, and toss well to coat.
4. In large salad bowl, combine lime juice, oil, and cilantro. Add greens, red bell pepper, and avocado, and toss well.
5. Top salad mix with chicken. Place toasted tortilla wedges around edge of salad bowl.

**MAKES 2 SERVINGS**

**Per serving:** *451 cal, 38 g pro, 30 g carb, 21.7 g fat, 4.2 g sat fat, 93 mg chol, 10 g fiber, 241 mg sodium*

## DINNER
- 6 oz trout fillet (grilled or broiled)
- 2 c broccoli and 1 tsp minced garlic, sautéed in 2 tsp olive oil
- 3/4 c brown rice

## POSTWORKOUT SNACK
- Strawberry Whey Shake (see page 18)

**DAY 2 TOTAL**
Protein 129 g
Carbohydrates 180 g
Fat 54 g
Saturated Fat 13 g
Cholesterol 242 mg
Fiber 38 g
Sodium 668 mg

# Plan C

Meal plans made for Cardio (C) days focus on low–glycemic index carbohydrates, such as oatmeal, bulgur, whole wheat, and chickpeas, from breakfast through dinner. The carbs in these foods slowly convert to glucose in the blood, so you won't get energy-sapping blood sugar spikes and dips throughout the day.

The payoff: plenty of fuel for sustaining a cardio workout and possibly better appetite control and less hunger. (A and B days have their share of low-GI carbs too, but Cardio days have about double the number.)

 **Day 1**

### BREAKFAST
- ¹/₂ c cooked oatmeal with ¹/₂ banana, sliced, and a dash of nutmeg; top with 1 tsp brown sugar and 2 Tbsp walnuts
- 1 c fat-free milk

### MIDMORNING SNACK
- 6 oz low-fat plain yogurt mixed with 1 tsp honey and ¹/₂ banana, sliced

### LUNCH
- 2 oz lean roast beef (such as Healthy Choice) tossed with 3 c watercress, ¹/₂ c rinsed and drained canned chickpeas, and a dressing of 1 Tbsp prepared horseradish, 1 Tbsp reduced-fat mayo, 1 tsp olive oil, and 1 tsp vinegar
- 100-calorie portion of trans-free whole grain crackers (such as 5 Triscuits)

### DINNER
- Whole Wheat Penne with Shrimp and Broccoli Rabe (see recipe on page 22)
- 100-calorie serving of dark chocolate (about 3/4 oz)

**DAY 1 TOTAL**
Protein 93 g
Carbohydrates 190 g
Fat 57 g
Saturated Fat 14 g
Cholesterol 231 mg
Fiber 28 g
Sodium 1,417 mg

# Whole Wheat Penne with Shrimp and Broccoli Rabe

PREP TIME: 7 MINUTES
COOKING TIME: 18 MINUTES

- 1 bunch (about 1 lb) broccoli rabe or Broccolini, cut into 3" lengths
- 8 oz whole wheat penne
- 4 Tbsp olive oil
- 1 lb med uncooked shrimp, peeled and deveined
- 2 tsp minced garlic
- 1/4–1/2 tsp red-pepper flakes
- 1/3 c seafood broth or reduced-sodium chicken broth
- 1/2 c chopped fresh basil
- 1/3 c grated Parmesan cheese

1. Bring 4 quarts of water to a boil in large pot over high heat. Add broccoli rabe, and cook until crisp-tender, about 1½ minutes. Remove with slotted spoon or tongs, and plunge into cold water. Drain, and set aside.

2. In same water, prepare pasta per package directions.

3. Meanwhile, heat 2 tablespoons of the oil over medium heat in large, heavy-bottomed pan. Place shrimp in pan in single layer. Cook, stirring once or twice, until shrimp are pink and just cooked through, about 2 minutes. With slotted spoon or tongs, transfer shrimp to medium bowl, and set aside.

4. Add remaining 2 tablespoons oil to pan, and sauté garlic over medium heat 30 seconds. Add red-pepper flakes and broccoli rabe, and sauté until soft but not soggy, about 2 minutes. Add shrimp, broth, and basil, and heat through, about 1 minute.

5. Drain pasta, and transfer to large serving bowl. Toss with cheese. Add shrimp and broccoli rabe mixture, and toss. Serve immediately.

**MAKES 4 SERVINGS**

**Per serving:** *548 cal, 41 g pro, 48 g carb, 20 g fat, 3.6 g sat fat, 180 mg chol, 10 g fiber, 407 mg sodium*

## ■ Day 2

### BREAKFAST
- 1 toasted whole wheat English muffin (such as Thomas' Hearty Grains) spread with 1 1/2 Tbsp peanut or almond butter and 2 tsp honey or jam
- 1 c fat-free milk
- 1 orange

### LUNCH
- 2 c lentil soup, heated with 2 c fresh spinach (choose a soup with less than 500 mg of sodium per cup, such as Progresso 99% Fat Free or Tabatchnick [frozen] Tuscany Lentil)
- 100-calorie serving of trans-free whole grain crackers (such as 5 Triscuits)
- 1/2 c carrot sticks or baby carrots

### AFTERNOON SNACK
- 1 small apple and 1 oz reduced-fat Cheddar cheese

### DINNER
- Bulgur with Pine Nuts (see recipe on page 24) with 3/4 c skinless cooked chicken and 1/3 c rinsed and drained canned chickpeas
- Salad of 3 plum tomatoes, sliced; 1 Tbsp chopped parsley; 1 scallion, sliced or chopped; 1 tsp olive oil; spritz of lemon; and salt and pepper to taste
- Mango Treat (see recipe below)

**DAY 2 TOTAL**
Protein 91 g
Carbohydrates 229 g
Fat 48 g
Saturated Fat 10 g
Cholesterol 105 mg
Fiber 40 g
Sodium 1,866 mg

# Mango Treat
PREP TIME: 3 MINUTES

      4  oz low-fat vanilla yogurt
    1/2  c mango sorbet
      4  raspberries (garnish)

Place yogurt in bowl, top with sorbet, and garnish with raspberries.

### MAKES 1 SERVING
**Per Serving:** 189 cal, 5 g pro, 40 g carb, 1.7 g fat, 1 g sat fat, 0 mg chol, 1 g fiber, 76 mg sodium

# Bulgur with Pine Nuts

PREP TIME: 3 MINUTES
COOKING TIME: 30 MINUTES

- ½ c coarse bulgur (not the fine bulgur used for tabbouleh)
- 1 c reduced-sodium chicken broth
- 4 Tbsp chopped green and red bell peppers
- 2 Tbsp pine nuts
- 2 Tbsp chopped parsley
  Green leaf lettuce (optional)

1. Add bulgur to broth in medium pot, and bring to a boil over high heat. Reduce heat to low, cover, and cook until bulgur is tender, 20 to 25 minutes.
2. Meanwhile, in nonstick skillet coated with cooking spray, sauté peppers over medium heat until soft, about 6 minutes. Toast nuts in small skillet over medium heat until golden brown, about 3 minutes. Stir frequently to prevent burning.
3. When bulgur is cooked, let stand 5 minutes, transfer to plate, and toss with peppers, nuts, and parsley. Serve over lettuce, if desired.

**MAKES 2 SERVINGS**

**Per serving:** *182 cal, 6 g pro, 28 g carb, 6.2 g fat, 0.5 g sat fat, 0 mg chol, 7 g fiber, 56 mg sodium*

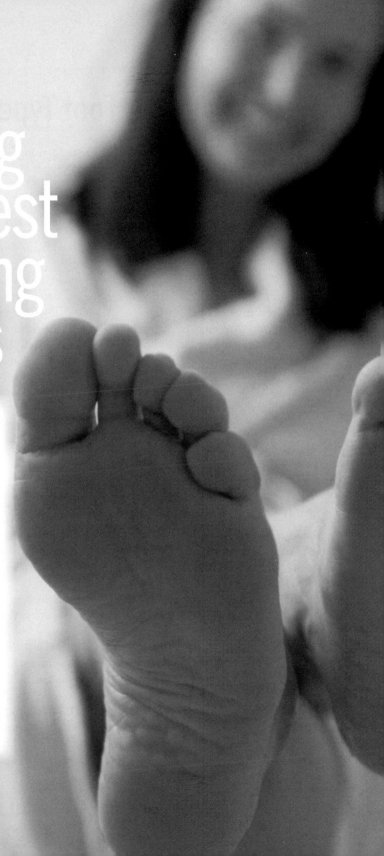

# CHAPTER 3

# buying the best walking shoes

C hances are, you have a closetful of shoes— pumps, flats, boots, and sandals for every outfit and occasion. Maybe you even have a pair of ballet slippers or bowling shoes from years ago. But unless you own a good pair of walking shoes—and they're still in great shape—you're going to have to do some shopping.

# Determining Your Foot Type

There's more to a good fit than just size. For a shoe to fit properly, it has to match the flexibility of your feet. You can easily determine this on your own by using this test.

## ■ Ruler Test

Flexibility refers to whether your feet are rigid, neutral, or flexible. To find out, do the following.

1. Sit in a chair, with one foot resting across the opposite knee. Measure the elevated foot from the heel to the tip of the longest toe (usually your big toe) by holding a ruler against the sole. Be careful not to press on the ruler, as that will skew the measurement. Write down the number, and then repeat this step with your other foot.

2. Lay the ruler on the floor, and stand on it with one foot. Measure from the heel to the tip of the longest toe. Write down the number, then switch feet and repeat.

3. Determine your foot type based on these descriptions.

- If the measurements taken when seated and when standing are about the same, your feet are rigid.
- If the measurements differ by about $1/8$ inch, your feet are neutral.
- If the measurements differ by about $1/4$ inch, your feet are flexible.

## ■ Follow Your Own Footprint

Armed with your foot type, you're ready to do some shoe shopping.

Go to a respected athletic-shoe store where a skilled salesperson can size up your feet, answer questions, and help you select and try on shoes, says Suki Munsell, PhD, director of the Dynamic Health and Fitness Institute in Corte Madera, California. Then, to save money on replacement pairs, you can go to a discount store and buy the same shoe for less money.

To make sure that a shoe is appropriate for you, look for features recommended for your foot type.

**FLEXIBLE** Of the three foot types, a flexible foot is the most complicated and most difficult to fit. It absorbs shock well because it's so mobile, but that mobility tends to make it unstable. Your foot rolls in too much (overpronates) when you walk. It changes one whole size when bearing weight. It also tends to be flat and have a low instep.

You don't need a lot of cushioning, but you do need a lot of arch support. You also need a low heel, which will do a better job of stabilizing your foot. You may feel most comfortable in a shoe with a straight last (bottom of shoe), as your foot tends to flatten and straighten out when you walk.

**NEUTRAL** Your foot is well-balanced, and it's the easiest type to fit. A neutral foot has normal mobility, which means it lengthens or spreads about half a shoe size when bearing weight (when you stand up, for example). It rolls on the ground, or pronates, almost perfectly. It absorbs shock well and has good stability. You can get by with less support, although a little extra won't hurt either. For a neutral foot, a shoe with a semicurved last (bottom of shoe) should fit well. You'll do well in soft, as well as supportive, shoes.

**RIGID** A rigid foot tends to have a high arch. It's stable, but it doesn't handle impact well. Your foot rolls inward very little during walking (underpronates) and is very stiff, so it doesn't absorb shock very well. (Flexibility allows your foot to become loose to absorb the impact with the ground.)

For this foot type, you need a shoe that is very well cushioned, because your arch is not going to flex and provide much cushioning for you. You also need an upper that has a lot of volume, or space to accommodate your high instep. You may have tight Achilles tendons (at the backs of your ankles), so you'll want your shoe to have a bit of a heel. Your foot will tend to curve, so look for a shoe that does likewise.

**TIP**

*Burning pain in the toes or in the ball of your foot could mean that you need roomier shoes. A visit to a podiatrist is also in order. You may have Morton's neuroma, a condition that can quickly be exacerbated. Other symptoms include tingling, numbness, or pain that radiates to surrounding areas. It may feel as if you're treading on a marble. The pain generally gets worse when wearing shoes or walking. Night pain is rare.*

*Morton's neuroma commonly occurs between the bases of the third and fourth toes. It's up to 10 times more common in women than men, possibly because it can be caused by wearing narrow, high shoes or even shoes that are too flat.*

*To feel better, make sure that your walking shoe is roomy in the toe box and has a low heel and a soft sole. Limit your time spent hoofing it in heels; if you must wear them, travel to work or a social event in comfier shoes and then slip on the more stylish pair. Over-the-counter insoles or pads that relieve pressure and absorb shock may help too. About 80% of people find relief from these steps. If pain interferes with daily activities, ask your doctor about corticosteroid injections to reduce swelling and inflammation.*

# Shoe-Shopping Savvy

To find your ideal match, you need to know when, where, and how to shop. Just follow these guidelines, and you'll be sure to get a great fit.

**Be a PM shopper.** Search for shoes at the end of the day, when your feet have swollen to their largest size.

**Maximize your options.** Go to a store that carries a wide variety of brands and styles so that you have the best chance of finding the right shoes.

**Get some advice.** Tell the salesperson your foot type and how often and how far you'll be walking.

**Check your size.** Ask to have your feet measured, if possible. As you get older, your feet tend to flatten out, which may affect your shoe size.

**Prepare for sticker shock.** Expect to pay between $55 and $85 for a good-quality, good-fitting pair of walking shoes. If the price seems high, consider the cost of an appointment with a podiatrist or orthopedist. You're worth the expense, and so are your shoes. Once you've selected a pair, you can go to other stores to see if you can get the same brand and style for less. Keep your eyes peeled for sales and discounts.

**Wear your walking socks.** Some styles are really thick, so you may need to choose a shoe that's a half-size larger than you normally wear to accommodate them. Speaking of socks, don't skimp on them. Next to your shoes, your socks are your most important piece of walking gear. The wrong pair of socks can ruin the feel of a great pair of shoes. Fortunately, there are now socks on the market just for walkers. Many have extra padding in the heel and ball of the foot. Try a variety of brands until you find what feels right for you. For more information about socks, see page 42.

**Leave some breathing room.** When you try on shoes, make sure there's plenty of space—at least one finger's width—beyond the end of your longest toe (usually the big toe). Measure this space when you're standing up rather than sitting down. Ideally, you should have someone else measure for you.

**Take a long test drive.** Spend time in the shoes. Walk around the store. If you're in a mall, ask if you can take a few laps around. The shoes should feel great; never buy a pair that you have to break in.

**T I P**

*If your shoes tend to get wet when you walk, invest in two pairs. This way, you can alternate between them, allowing each pair to fully dry, and extend the life of your shoes. If you have only one pair, stuff newspaper inside your wet shoes to help soak up moisture faster, so they might be dry by the next day. Don't put wet leather shoes near heat; drying them too fast can cause them to shrink or crack.*

# Lacing Up Properly

Foot characteristics such as a narrow heel or low arch can affect the fit of your shoes, says Tom Brunick, director of The Athlete's Foot store's research and development center in Naperville, Illinois. For a better fit, try these fancy lacing techniques. (The shoelaces are two-toned for clarification.)

### NARROW HEEL

Lace normally until the last set of holes. Instead of lacing across the shoe, pull the laces up toward the ankle to thread down through the last hole on each side, thus creating a loop by not pulling the lace all the way through. Cross the laces and thread through the loops, then tighten and tie.

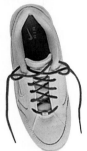

### LOW ARCH

Use crisscross lacing halfway up the shoe, then use the "loop lacing" technique (as done for the narrow heel, above) for the remaining holes.

### HIGH ARCH

Make your first crisscross as usual, then thread straight up the next several holes on each side. Crisscross the last set of holes.

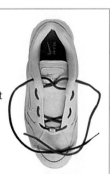

### WIDE FOOT

Thread straight up the first two or three sets of holes on each side. Start crisscrossing once you're past the forefoot.

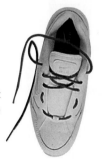

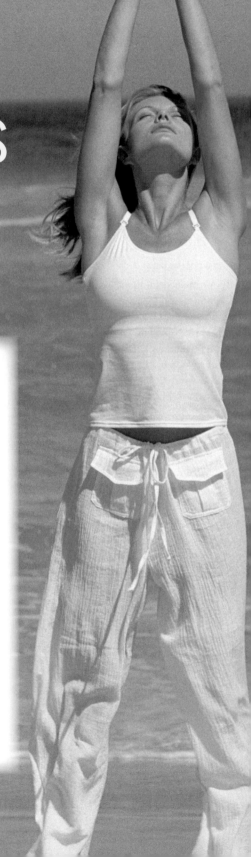

# CHAPTER 4
# stretches for walkers

Feel your best by warming up and cooling down properly for every workout. To begin, spend 5 minutes walking at an easy pace to get your muscles and joints ready for more vigorous activity. (If you want to stretch at the beginning of your workout, do so after you have warmed up.) Then conclude your workout with a cool-down and stretch. Slow your pace for the last 5 minutes to bring your heart rate and breathing back to normal. With your muscles warmed up, now is the best time to stretch them out and increase your flexibility, which often decreases as we get older and become less active. And ending with these feel-good stretches will make you more likely to exercise tomorrow.

## CHEST

Stand with your feet about shoulder width apart, and grasp your hands behind your back, fingers intertwined and palms facing in. Keeping your chest lifted and shoulders down, squeeze your shoulder blades, and gently lift your arms as high as comfortable. Don't arch your back. Hold while you take three deep breaths, and then release.

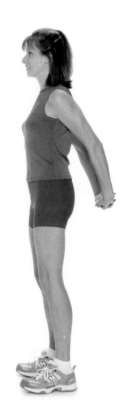

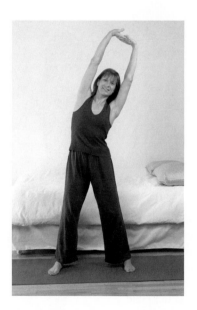

## SIDE

Stand with your feet wider than shoulder width apart. Clasp your hands overhead, pressing your palms toward the ceiling. Lift up, and then bend slightly to your left. You should feel a stretch down the right side of your torso. Hold for three deep breaths, and then release. Repeat to the other side.

## CALF

Bend your right leg, and place your left foot about 2 feet behind you, pressing your heel into the floor. Your left leg should be straight, and you should feel a stretch in your left calf. Hold while you take three deep breaths, and then release. Switch legs, and repeat.

## HAMSTRINGS

From the calf stretch position, step your back foot in 6 to 12 inches, and bend that leg. Straighten your front leg, bringing your toes off the floor, and sit back, shifting your weight onto your back foot. Don't lock your front knee. Place your hands on your bent leg for support. You should feel a stretch in the back of your straight leg. Hold while you take three deep breaths, and then release. Switch legs, and repeat.

## QUADRICEPS

Standing with your feet together, bend your left leg behind you, bringing that foot toward your buttocks. Grasp your left foot with your left hand, and tuck your hips under so that you feel a stretch in the front of your left thigh and hip. (You can hold on to a chair or a wall with your right hand for balance if you need to.) Hold while you take three deep breaths, and then release. Switch legs, and repeat.

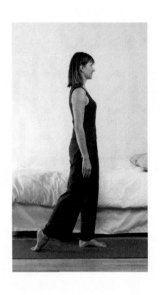

## SHIN

Step your right foot back about 6 inches and point your toes back so that the top of your foot rests on the floor. Bending your left knee, press down into your right foot so that you feel a stretch in your right shin. Hold for three deep breaths, and then release. Switch legs, and repeat.

## HIP

Sit on the edge of your bed, chair, or bench, and place your left foot on your right knee. Your right hand should be on top of your left ankle, and your left hand on top of your left knee. Keeping your back straight, bend at the hips and lean forward. You should feel a stretch in your left hip. For a deeper stretch, gently push on your left knee. Hold for three deep breaths, and then release. Switch legs, and repeat.

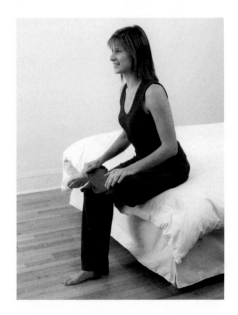

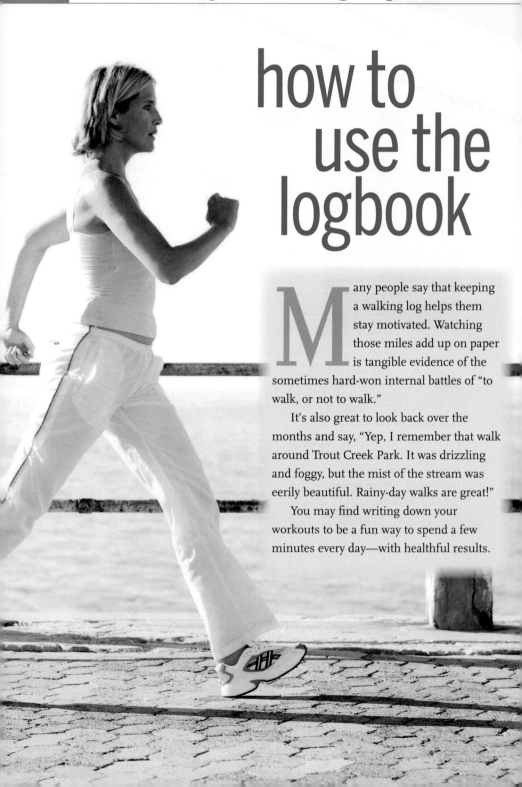

# how to use the logbook

**M**any people say that keeping a walking log helps them stay motivated. Watching those miles add up on paper is tangible evidence of the sometimes hard-won internal battles of "to walk, or not to walk."

It's also great to look back over the months and say, "Yep, I remember that walk around Trout Creek Park. It was drizzling and foggy, but the mist of the stream was eerily beautiful. Rainy-day walks are great!"

You may find writing down your workouts to be a fun way to spend a few minutes every day—with healthful results.

Whether you're an experienced walker or just starting out, the logbook and journal are your daily reminders to get out there and do it!

Start your journal by developing your personalized workouts and walking plans. In chapter 1, you learned all about the A-B-C Walking Plan. Now it's time to pick a program that appeals to you. Pencil your planned activities into the shaded A-B-C Daily Plan section of the logbook. When that day arrives, just head out the door, pull out an exercise mat, turn on the treadmill, or fire up the TV and pop in the exercise DVD, and get going. At the end of your session, you can record when and where you worked out, how long it took you, the miles you covered or the steps you took, and at what pace.

## RECORD YOUR THOUGHTS

In the "Notes" section, be sure to record not just how you felt physically on the walk, but also how you felt mentally. If you walked alone, with a friend, with your spouse, or with your dog, note that too.

There are several ways you can enhance your record keeping and make it more motivating. Keep track of your daily weight or your resting pulse (taken before you get out of bed in the morning). What's your time for a mile? How do your feet feel?

Another great thing to do is record your routes. If you enjoy walking the same route, what changes do you see from day to day? Increase your powers of observation. If you alternate routes, document them so that you can go back there or take a partner to the best routes.

## LOOK FOR PATTERNS

For days when you're having trouble getting off the couch, flip through your journal and see all the miles you've logged. Reviewing your progress can be a great motivator.

To make your walks more rewarding look through your comments from time to time to see if patterns emerge: What made your walks easier—walking with your friend? What made them harder—walking with your dog, who likes to stop and sniff everything? Then use this information when planning future walks.

## CELEBRATE YOUR SUCCESS

As you near the finish line in week 4, you'll be able to give yourself a pat on the back by seeing how far you've come.

The following example shows how you might fill out a day of your logbook.

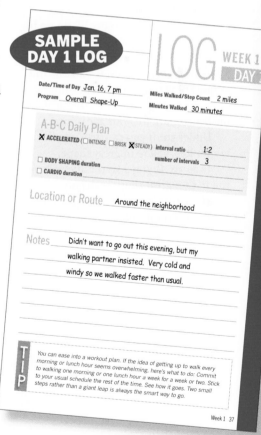

**SAMPLE DAY 1 LOG**

LOG WEEK 1 DAY 1

Date/Time of Day Jan. 16, 7 pm
Program Overall Shape-Up
Miles Walked/Step Count 2 miles
Minutes Walked 30 minutes

A-B-C Daily Plan
X ACCELERATED (☐ INTENSE ☐ BRISK X STEADY) interval ratio 1:2
☐ BODY SHAPING duration number of intervals 3
☐ CARDIO duration

Location or Route Around the neighborhood

Notes Didn't want to go out this evening, but my walking partner insisted. Very cold and windy so we walked faster than usual.

TIP You can ease into a workout plan. If the idea of getting up to walk every morning or lunch hour seems overwhelming, here's what to do: Commit to walking one morning or one lunch hour a week for a week or two. Stick to your usual schedule the rest of the time. See how it goes. Two small steps rather than a giant leap is always the smart way to go.

Week 1 37

# CHAPTER 5

# Week 1

Weight _____

# DAY 1

## FOCUS ON FITNESS

Before you start the A-B-C Walking Plan, take this test developed by James Rippe, MD, author of *Dr. James Rippe's Complete Book of Fitness Walking,* to assess your current fitness level.

Find a flat 1-mile route. Warm up by walking at an easy pace for 5 minutes and stretching your calves and hamstrings. Then time yourself as you walk the mile as quickly as you can without running out of steam. Compare your results against the benchmark for your age group.

**Under 30:** If you can walk a mile in 13 minutes, you're in great shape.

**30 to 39:** Doing a 14-minute mile puts you in the "great shape" category.

**40 to 49:** Cover a mile in just under 15 minutes (14 minutes, 42 seconds), and

you're at the top level of fitness for your age group.

**50 to 69:** Completing a 15-minute mile is excellent.

**70 or over:** If you can walk a mile in 18 minutes and 18 seconds, you're very fit for your age.

If you exceed the ideal time for your age group, you're not in the best shape aerobically. But don't worry—just keep walking. Regular, consistent exercise can improve your fitness and decrease your time.

If you're new to walking, however, build up your time and mileage gradually. After all, you want your feet to toughen up and your muscles to get used to the exertion. You may not actually hurt yourself, but if you feel stiff and sore because you did too much too quickly, it may keep you from going out again.

Date/Time of Day _____    Miles Walked/Step Count _____

Program _____    Minutes Walked _____

## A-B-C Daily Plan

☐ **ACCELERATED** (☐INTENSE ☐BRISK ☐STEADY) **interval ratio** _____

**number of intervals** _____

☐ **BODY SHAPING duration** _____

☐ **CARDIO duration** _____

## Location or Route _____

_____

_____

## Notes _____

_____

_____

_____

_____

_____

_____

**TIP**

*You can ease into a workout plan. If the idea of getting up to walk every morning or lunch hour seems overwhelming, here's what to do: Commit to walking one morning or one lunch hour a week for a week or two. Stick to your usual schedule the rest of the time. See how it goes. Two small steps rather than a giant leap is always the smart way to go.*

# DAY 2

## TIMING IS EVERYTHING

Most experts will tell you that if you want to be consistent, your best bet is to walk first thing in the morning. By getting it out of the way early, there's less chance that your workout will be sidelined by other obligations that arise over the course of a day.

If this works for you, fantastic. An early-morning walk can be a great start to a productive day. By the time you finish your workout, your energy level will be up, and you'll feel relaxed and energized. Plus, if you get out the door early enough, you'll beat the early-morning commuters. That means there's less traffic and less car exhaust to deal with.

But don't force yourself to become a morning person if you'd rather sleep in. You need to find a time to exercise that suits your schedule and your lifestyle. Choosing the right time to walk can make committing to an exercise program much easier.

For you, lunch may be the perfect time to walk, especially if you work outside your home and you have young children or other responsibilities that keep you from getting out of the house early in the morning or after dinner. For working parents, a lunch-hour workout can seem like a mini-vacation. It's a great opportunity for you to destress.

One word of advice, though: Try to walk first and eat lunch afterward. That way, you can travel at a brisk pace without aggravating your digestive system. And you may find that you're less hungry by the time you get back—a bonus if you're trying to lose weight. If you're starving by lunchtime, eat a small snack (a piece of fruit, 1/2 bagel with peanut butter, yogurt, or cheese on whole grain crackers) about an hour before your workout, to tide you over until you've finished your workout.

If you and your spouse like to exercise together, you may prefer to take after-dinner walks. They're a wonderful opportunity for the two of you to spend time together and to discuss the day's events away from the dishes, the telephone, and the TV. Just plan on going at a leisurely pace. When you walk after a meal, your body is putting all of its energy into digesting food. If you walk too fast, you may end up with cramps or indigestion.

Depending on your schedule, you may have to do your walking just before bedtime. You can revel in the quiet of the evening. Keep in mind that walking at night isn't for everyone. While some say that it's the perfect nightcap, others find it too stimulating. Safety is an issue too (see page 66). Experiment to find out whether it's right for you.

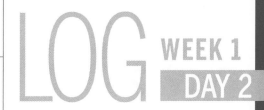

**Date/Time of Day** _____

**Miles Walked/Step Count** _____

**Program** _____

**Minutes Walked** _____

## A-B-C Daily Plan

☐ **ACCELERATED** (☐ INTENSE ☐ BRISK ☐ STEADY) **interval ratio** _____

**number of intervals** _____

☐ **BODY SHAPING duration** _____

☐ **CARDIO duration** _____

## Location or Route _____

_____

_____

## Notes _____

_____

_____

_____

_____

_____

_____

_____

_____

_____

**T I P**

*If your choice of walking terrain is between a concrete sidewalk and an asphalt- or tar-paved road, choose the latter because it's softer. If the road slants toward the curb, reverse the direction you walk every couple of days to avoid injuries resulting from walking on an uneven surface.*

# DAY 3

## FIND THE FAT IN YOUR SCHEDULE

"The number-one reason people stop exercising is lack of time," says Harold Kohl, PhD, an epidemiologist with the Physical Activity and Health Branch of the Centers for Disease Control and Prevention (CDC). For busy people, getting at least 30 minutes of moderate-intensity exercise 5 or more days a week might as well be suggesting racewalking to the moon. Kohl says an attitude adjustment is in order. "Take a hard look at your day and figure out where you can substitute activity for inactivity," he says. "Think about exercise the way you think about substituting low-fat food for high-fat food." Any walking is better than none, he continues. "The key is to look for opportunities to be active in ways that aren't necessarily planned or structured. In other words, look beyond the stuff we typically think of as exercise." Once you adopt Kohl's thinking, opportunities for activity appear everywhere.

**Up your downtime.** Walk in place or do some squats while catching up on phone calls to friends or family. For yard work, choose a push mower over a power one. If you're waiting at the school-bus stop, breeze up and down the block (keeping the stop in sight) until the bus pulls into view. Got mail? Scout out a drop box a 10-minute walk away. And when you get stuck at the airport, don't take the wait sitting down. Instead, hike through the terminal.

**Leave the stands.** Do you spend time schlepping your offspring to sports events? Never just sit and watch. Do laps around the field to give yourself a workout as well as several vantage points to view the action.

**Look for bite-size exercise.** Instead of waiting until you have a free half hour, dissect your goal into bite-size nuggets. Think of your daily exercise allotment as three 10-minute jaunts, six 5-minute spurts, or even fifteen 2-minute quickies (roughly equivalent to the number of commercial breaks in an evening spent watching television). "Studies show that you burn the same number of calories whether you exercise all at once or in short bursts," says Liz Neporent, *Prevention* contributing editor and author of *Fitness Walking for Dummies*.

**Use your indoor track.** Walking laps around the house may sound dizzying, but it works for women pressed for time or caring for young children, says Neporent. "You can walk in place while you're waiting for water to boil or watching television," she says. "The average person walks a mile in 15 to 20 minutes, and it doesn't matter if you do it moving or standing in place." To make stationary walking more of a challenge, Neporent suggests adding some high knee lifts and big arm swings.

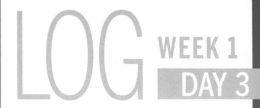

**Date/Time of Day** _____    **Miles Walked/Step Count** _____

**Program** _____    **Minutes Walked** _____

## A-B-C Daily Plan

☐ **ACCELERATED** (☐INTENSE ☐BRISK ☐STEADY)  **interval ratio** _____

**number of intervals** _____

☐ **BODY SHAPING duration** _____

☐ **CARDIO duration** _____

## Location or Route _____

_____

_____

## Notes _____

_____

_____

_____

_____

_____

**TIP**

*Walk, don't wait. Whenever you have to wait—for a restaurant table, doctor's appointment, child's music lesson, or soccer practice—don't just sit there, walk! (Let the receptionist know you'll be circling the block, checking in at each lap.)*

# DAY 4

## DRESS FOR SUCCESS

Next to shoes, your socks are your most important piece of walking gear. A lousy pair of socks can make a great pair of shoes feel absolutely awful. On the other hand, an okay pair of shoes can feel a lot more tolerable when they're worn over a fantastic pair of socks.

Thorlo was probably the first company to realize that folks would appreciate a little cushioning in their socks since human feet lose their fatty padding as they get older. Many stores carry dizzying displays of socks in all brands, colors, sizes, and styles. Some are thick; some are thin. Some support your arch; others pad your bunion. Many footwear manufacturers offer socks bearing the same brand names as their shoes.

Try a variety of brands and styles until you find one that you really like. Then buy a whole bunch, so you always have a clean pair waiting for you.

When you're going for a long walk— say, more than 4 miles—you may want to carry an extra pair of socks with you. Then if your feet get hot or wet, just change socks. You'll feel totally refreshed and revitalized.

Now that you have your feet properly attired, what about the rest of you? Let the temperature outside be your guide when you're deciding what to wear.

For warm-weather walking, you need a pair of comfortable shorts that won't ride up the inside of your legs, such as stretch shorts similar to those worn for cycling. On top, a cotton-polyester blend T-shirt is fine. It will be softer than a 100% cotton shirt, and it won't shrink.

For cooler weather, sweatpants or stretch pants are great. Choose a fabric that breathes and wicks away sweat. Make sure that your pants allow for a full range of motion. Avoid those that are too tight around the waist. You need to breathe. On top, you may want a long-sleeved T-shirt and a lightweight jacket, depending on the temperature.

Thanks to an array of high-tech textiles, you can be warm and dry and still have freedom of movement in winter. New fabrics insulate, block the wind, and wick away moisture without bulk or heaviness.

Even though new fabrics are lightweight, the layered look is still your best bet. That way, you can adjust your attire as you go, according to the weather and your level of activity.

• For the innermost layer (the one closest to your skin), choose light garments made from a synthetic fabric such as polypropylene, which wicks perspiration away from your body.

• Top this off with an insulating layer—a sweater, a sweatshirt, or a fleece pullover—for warmth.

• For the outermost layer, or shell, you want a garment that protects you from wind and rain. The fabric should be waterproof, as opposed to water resistant (which is designed to keep you dry in a light mist). It should also be breathable— meaning that it allows water vapor to escape without actually letting water in.

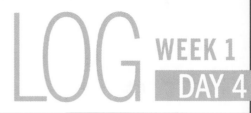

# LOG WEEK 1 DAY 4

**Date/Time of Day** _____     **Miles Walked/Step Count** _____

**Program** _____     **Minutes Walked** _____

## A-B-C Daily Plan

☐ **ACCELERATED** (☐ INTENSE  ☐ BRISK  ☐ STEADY)  **interval ratio** _____

                                                                     **number of intervals** _____

☐ **BODY SHAPING duration** _____

☐ **CARDIO duration** _____

## Location or Route _____

_____

_____

## Notes _____

_____

_____

_____

_____

_____

_____

_____

_____

_____

_____

# DAY 5

## PERFECT YOUR WALK

Here are the key points for good walking posture. To check your form, have a friend watch you walk, or walk on a treadmill in front of a mirror.

- **Stand tall:** Imagine a wire attached to the top of your head, pulling it upward.
- **Head:** Keep your chin up and your ears in line with your shoulders.
- **Eyes:** Look 6 to 10 feet in front.
- **Shoulders:** Keep them relaxed, down, and back.
- **Chest:** Imagine that there's a headlight in your breastbone—shine it forward, not down on the ground.
- **Arms:** Relax and swing from the shoulders. Pump your arms forward and back; don't "chicken-wing" them across your body.
- **Elbows:** Bend them at 85- to 90-degree angles.
- **Hands:** Cup them loosely. Pump forward, not across your body.
- **Abdominals:** Keep them firm.
- **Back:** Stand straight; don't arch.
- **Pelvis:** Tuck slightly by pulling your belly button back toward your spine.
- **Hips:** Swivel them.
- **Knees:** Keep them soft and pointing forward.

- **Feet:** Point your toes forward, keeping your feet parallel to each other.
- **Front foot:** Plant your heel first; don't let your foot fall inward or outward.
- **Back foot:** Roll forward, pressing into the centerline of your foot; push off with your toes.

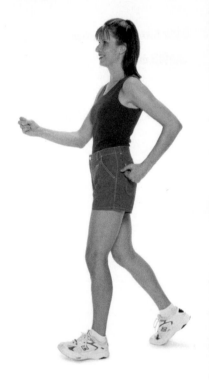

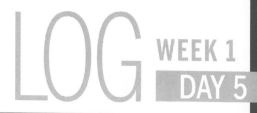

Date/Time of Day _____    Miles Walked/Step Count _____

Program _____    Minutes Walked _____

## A-B-C Daily Plan

☐ **ACCELERATED** (☐ INTENSE  ☐ BRISK  ☐ STEADY) **interval ratio** _____

**number of intervals** _____

☐ **BODY SHAPING duration** _____

☐ **CARDIO duration** _____

## Location or Route _____

_____

_____

## Notes _____

_____

_____

_____

_____    **T**
                                        **I**   To stand up tall, bend your
_____     **P**   left arm behind your waist
                                                 and grab your right arm at
_____             the elbow. This simple move
                                                 pulls your shoulders back and
_____             down (where they belong).
                                                 Hold for about 10 seconds,
_____             and then switch arms. Do two
                                                 or three times throughout
_____             your walk.

# DAY 6

## DRINK UP

Dehydration is a real downer. If you haven't had enough to drink, you can feel light-headed, headachy, dizzy, and confused and can have increased heart and breathing rates. "Even a small amount of water loss can impair your ability to perform at your best and feel good about exercising," says Christine Rosenbloom, PhD, RD, associate professor of nutrition at Georgia State University.

When you exercise, don't wait until you feel thirsty to imbibe: Drink 6 to 8 ounces of liquid before and after your walk. And sip something every 15 minutes during your workout.

But don't get waterlogged. Drinking too much water can result in a serious condition called hyponatremia (low sodium levels). At greatest risk are recreational athletes who take more than 4 hours to complete an event in hot, humid weather and those who take too many water breaks. Women appear to be more vulnerable than men.

Symptoms, which may not show up until hours after a long walk, include shortness of breath, vomiting, and headache. In severe cases, seizures,

coma, and death can follow if not treated immediately. Sport drinks and salty foods won't combat the problem; prevention is the key.

If you're walking for long periods of time, you need to assess your body's water needs during your training program, says John Cianca, MD, of Baylor College of Medicine in Houston.

1. Weigh yourself before you exercise.

2. Walk for 1 hour without drinking anything.

3. Stop, towel off, and step on the scale to weigh yourself again.

4. Drink 16 ounces of fluid for every pound lost during the hour.

This will give you a good idea of what you'll need to drink per hour for long walks.

---

**T I P**

*It's a good idea to create a backup plan for your exercise regime. Map out three walks of varying lengths—10, 20, and 30 minutes (Beginners, halve those times)—near your home, office, and child's school so you have several options on busy days.*

---

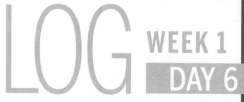

# LOG

Date/Time of Day _____  Miles Walked/Step Count _____

Program _____  Minutes Walked _____

## A-B-C Daily Plan

☐ **ACCELERATED** (☐ INTENSE ☐ BRISK ☐ STEADY)  **interval ratio** _____

**number of intervals** _____

☐ **BODY SHAPING duration** _____

☐ **CARDIO duration** _____

## Location or Route _____

_____

_____

## Notes _____

_____

_____

_____

_____

_____

_____

_____

_____

_____

_____

_____

# DAY 7

## COUNT ON A PEDOMETER

This handy gadget clips onto your waistband and detects the movement of your legs so it can count the number of steps you take. Then some pedometers multiply that number by the length of your stride, to get your mileage.

Because a pedometer registers leg movement, the way that you position it on your body is important. To count steps accurately, pedometers need to hang vertically from your waist, aligned over your knee. If you have a large belly, it can push your pedometer out at an angle, throwing off its accuracy. Don't let this discourage you; try attaching the pedometer to your front pocket for a more accurate reading.

If your pedometer tracks mileage, you'll need to input your stride length. Here's how to get an accurate measure.

1. Mark off a level 20-foot path.

2. Walk that distance, counting the number of steps you take. Give yourself room for a walking start, so you're using a relaxed, normal gait by the time you reach the marked-off section.

3. Divide the distance (20 feet) by the number of steps it takes you to walk that far. For example, if you took 10 steps, divide 20 by 10 for a stride length of 2 feet.

4. Repeat this process three times. Then use those results to calculate an average stride length.

5. Set your pedometer to that stride length, and go.

## TIP

*Walking on a soft surface like sand can burn 20 to 50% more calories than walking on a paved road, says Hermann J. Engels, PhD, professor of exercise science at Wayne State University in Detroit. Basically, the softer the surface, the more effort you have to put into each step, making you burn more calories.*

*Caution: All that hard work could lead to an injury. So ease into beach walking and keep your shoes on to protect your feet.*

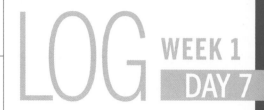

# LOG WEEK 1
## DAY 7

**Date/Time of Day** _____  **Miles Walked/Step Count** _____

**Program** _____  **Minutes Walked** _____

## A-B-C Daily Plan

☐ **ACCELERATED** (☐ INTENSE  ☐ BRISK  ☐ STEADY)  **interval ratio** _____

**number of intervals** _____

☐ **BODY SHAPING duration** _____

☐ **CARDIO duration** _____

## Location or Route _____

_____

_____

## Notes _____

_____

_____

_____

_____

_____

_____

_____

_____

_____

_____

_____

# CHAPTER 6

# Week 2

Weight _____

Pounds Lost _____

# DAY 1

## DON'T DRINK YOUR CALORIES

Some 10% to 14% of your daily calories don't come from food at all, according to the USDA. Instead, they sneak through in beverages that wash down those calorie-counted meals. While it's important to stay hydrated, some beverages can wreak havoc on your waistline. One caffe latte for breakfast, one can of soda at lunch, and a fruit smoothie snack can blow your daily budget by 550 calories!

While they're certainly tasty going down, liquid calories don't register on your appetite meter the way solid food does. In a study in which researchers asked 15 people to drink an extra 450 calories a day (the amount in three cans of soda), they gained weight. When they consumed the same number of additional calories from food, however, their weight didn't change.

They made up for the extra food by eating less throughout the day. But they didn't compensate for the drinks, thus adding 450 calories to their normal day's total.

And studies also have found that the more sweetened beverages people drink, the less likely they are to be getting enough essential vitamins and minerals, such as bone-building calcium and heart-protective folate.

Limit calorie-filled beverages, except for calcium-rich, low-fat or fat-free dairy or soy milk and antioxidant-rich tomato, orange, or Concord grape juice. Just keep tabs on how much you're drinking, or dilute the juice with sparkling water or diet lemon soda for a refreshing twist. Most of the time, stick to calorie-free beverages such as water, club soda, or unsweetened iced tea.

> **TIP**
>
> *Research suggests that antioxidants can help reduce the inflammation and stress that exercise puts on your body. To fully unlock their power, make sure you're eating enough good fats. Aim for two weekly servings of fish rich in omega-3s, such as salmon, tuna, mackerel, and sardines.*

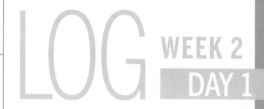

Date/Time of Day _____    Miles Walked/Step Count _____

Program _____    Minutes Walked _____

## A-B-C Daily Plan

☐ **ACCELERATED** (☐ INTENSE  ☐ BRISK  ☐ STEADY)  **interval ratio** _____

**number of intervals** _____

☐ **BODY SHAPING duration** _____

☐ **CARDIO duration** _____

## Location or Route _____

_____

_____

## Notes _____

_____

_____

_____

_____

_____

_____

_____

_____

_____

_____

# DAY 2

## WALK OFF POUNDS AND BOOST ENERGY

Samara Ferber didn't realize how out of shape she was until her first date with Kiff Rasmussen, the man who almost didn't become her fiancé. "We met online, and I lied about how much I weighed," explains Ferber, who had gradually put on 80 pounds since college. When their e-mail romance began about a year and a half ago, she weighed 230. She told Rasmussen 150.

To her mind, she didn't look noticeably different from a 150-pound woman. "I was in denial about my weight," Ferber says. "When we met, Kiff was really upset—not about the weight, but because I'd lied to him." He came around. They continued seeing each other. And Ferber, no longer in denial, signed up for Jenny Craig and began walking after work.

"At the beginning, I just aimed to get out and move," she explains. The first day, she decided she'd simply walk for a half hour around her neighborhood in Englewood, Colorado, a community that sits among the wooded foothills of the Rockies. "I did the half hour; then I measured the distance in my car and was surprised to see I'd gone over a mile," Ferber recalls, her voice rising with enthusiasm. "I thought, Wow! It was easier than I'd expected. I felt exhilarated because I'd actually done something fun and easy that I could do all the time."

Gradually (so it didn't become so difficult that it stopped being fun), Ferber picked up her pace and pushed her distance. A year later, she was walking 5-Ks. These days, she walks a 12-minute mile and is training for a triathlon. "I'll walk more than run it, since walking is easier on my knees," says Ferber, who's walking three times a week and biking and swimming once a week to prepare. Since she started walking, she's lost 70 pounds.

"I'm busy, but I fit walking in because it's crucial to my overall well-being," Ferber says. Without all that excess weight to tote around, she feels better and has more stamina. "It keeps me feeling strong so I can manage everything else that comes along."

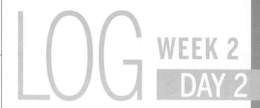
**Date/Time of Day** _____

**Program** _____

**Miles Walked/Step Count** _____

**Minutes Walked** _____

## A-B-C Daily Plan

☐ **ACCELERATED** (☐ INTENSE ☐ BRISK ☐ STEADY) **interval ratio** _____

**number of intervals** _____

☐ **BODY SHAPING duration** _____

☐ **CARDIO duration** _____

## Location or Route _____

_____

_____

## Notes _____

_____

_____

_____

_____

_____

_____

_____

_____

_____

_____

**T I P**

*As you walk, roll from heel to toe, pressing into the centerline of your foot, and push off with your toes. This technique automatically incorporates your hips and buttocks, creating a powerful stride that shapes your entire leg, tightens your butt, and trims your waistline.*

# DAY 3

## WHAT'S THE REAL TEMPERATURE?

Sometimes it's tough to tell when a nice, warm day is actually too hot for safe outdoor exercise. You've no doubt learned from experience that high humidity makes a high air temperature feel even more uncomfortable. The combination of humidity and air temperature is known as apparent temperature. And as it rises, so does your risk of heat exhaustion or heatstroke, which can be life threatening.

So when the mercury is rising, look up the day's apparent temperature on the chart below, and then check it against the recommendations that follow.

- **90°F and below:** Head for the great outdoors.
- **91° to 104°F:** Proceed with caution.
- **105° to 129°F:** Consider indoor options unless you're acclimated to these conditions.
- **130°F and above:** Stay indoors.

## HOT-WEATHER WORKOUT GUIDE

*To determine the apparent temperature on any given day, find the environmental temperature (that is, the temperature of the outside air) at the top of the chart and the relative humidity on the left-hand side. Then locate the number where the respective column and row meet. That's the apparent temperature.*

| | ENVIRONMENTAL TEMPERATURE (IN FAHRENHEIT) | | | | | | | |
|---|---|---|---|---|---|---|---|---|
| | 75° | 80° | 85° | 90° | 95° | 100° | 105° | 110° |
| **APPARENT TEMPERATURE (IN FAHRENHEIT)** | | | | | | | | |
| **0%** | 69 | 73 | 78 | 83 | 87 | 91 | 95 | 99 |
| **10%** | 70 | 75 | 80 | 85 | 90 | 95 | 100 | 105 |
| **20%** | 72 | 77 | 82 | 87 | 93 | 99 | 105 | 112 |
| **30%** | 73 | 78 | 84 | 90 | 96 | 104 | 113 | 123 |
| **40%** | 74 | 79 | 86 | 93 | 101 | 110 | 123 | 137 |
| **50%** | 75 | 81 | 88 | 96 | 107 | 120 | 135 | 150 |
| **60%** | 76 | 82 | 90 | 100 | 114 | 132 | 149 | |
| **70%** | 77 | 85 | 93 | 106 | 124 | 144 | | |
| **80%** | 78 | 86 | 97 | 113 | 136 | | | |
| **90%** | 79 | 88 | 102 | 122 | | | | |
| **100%** | 80 | 91 | 108 | | | | | |

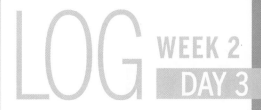

**Date/Time of Day** _____  **Miles Walked/Step Count** _____

**Program** _____  **Minutes Walked** _____

## A-B-C Daily Plan

☐ **ACCELERATED** (☐ INTENSE  ☐ BRISK  ☐ STEADY) **interval ratio** _____

**number of intervals** _____

☐ **BODY SHAPING duration** _____

☐ **CARDIO duration** _____

## Location or Route _____

_____

_____

## Notes _____

_____

_____

_____

_____

_____

_____

_____

_____

_____

# DAY 4

## DETERMINE YOUR PACE

The easiest way to gauge your speed without wearing a pedometer—or getting in your car and measuring mileage, which can be pretty difficult unless you walk along a street—is to count your number of steps per minute. You can use this number to calculate pace (how fast you cover a mile), based on an average stride length of 2 1/2 feet. (Stride length is the distance from the heel of one foot to the heel of the other foot when you're taking a step.) We've already done the math for you, and the results are below.

- 70 steps per minute equals 30 minutes per mile, or 2 miles per hour.
- 105 steps per minute equals 20 minutes per mile, or 3 miles per hour.
- 140 steps per minute equals 15 minutes per mile, or 4 miles per hour.

If you pay attention to your steps, after a while, you'll be able to estimate your pace fairly accurately without bothering to count. You'll just know what a 20-minute mile or a 15-minute mile feels like.

Here's another way to determine your pace. You may not think of your watch as walking gear. But it can become an indispensable part of your workout—and not just for showing you when it's time to turn around and head for home.

If you're walking on a measured course, you can time each mile of your workouts and use that to track improvements in your speed and strength. Plus, you get to know how it feels to walk at a certain pace.

Time yourself, and then match this to the speeds noted at the left. For example, if you cover a mile in 20 minutes, you're moving at a pace of 3 miles per hour.

If you cover a mile in 12 minutes, you're cruising at a pace of 5 miles per hour. As you might imagine, increasing your pace—going from a 20-minute mile to a 15-minute mile, for example—takes effort. At those speeds, you will make great strides in fitness and burn more calories.

> **TIP**
>
> *Hill walking burns up to 60% more calories than walking at the same pace on level ground—and it's great for firming your butt. If your area is flatter than day-old Coke, a treadmill with an incline setting will do the trick.*

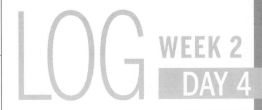

Date/Time of Day _____   Miles Walked/Step Count _____

Program _____   Minutes Walked _____

## A-B-C Daily Plan

☐ **ACCELERATED** (☐ INTENSE ☐ BRISK ☐ STEADY) **interval ratio** _____

**number of intervals** _____

☐ **BODY SHAPING duration** _____

☐ **CARDIO duration** _____

## Location or Route _____

_____

_____

## Notes _____

_____

_____

_____

_____

_____

_____

_____

_____

_____

_____

# DAY 5

## THINK YOURSELF FITTER

When you're trying to get in shape, your mind can be both your best friend and your worst enemy. At a moment's notice, the strong inner voice that encouraged you to exercise or cut back on fat can turn cruel, undermining your weight loss efforts with negative emotions and an endless stream of criticism. You tend to achieve what you focus on, so when negativity gets you down, you need to fight back—fast.

**Muzzle that inner critic.** A friend who constantly told you how fat you looked probably wouldn't be your friend for very long. So if you wouldn't put up with that kind of abuse from others, don't put up with it from yourself. Every time you hear your inner critic, stop what you're doing. Then think of something to encourage yourself, just as you'd try to encourage a friend. Say to yourself, "Okay, my body isn't as thin and fit as I'd like, but I'm working on it. I'm making progress."

**Banish all-or-nothing thinking.** Just because you don't have 45 minutes to work out doesn't mean that you should skip exercising entirely. After I had my son, I had to tell myself this over and over again. My workouts became more casual. Forget changing into exercise clothes; I'd just slip on my sneakers for a quick walk around the block with him on my shoulders. Or I'd go up and down the steps an extra time whenever I used them at work. Doing something is better than doing nothing.

> **TIP**
>
> *To improve balance and coordination, build bone, and burn fat faster, add some playfulness to your walk. Hop on or off curbs; zigzag between pavement, grass, and dirt; and attack head-on whatever sloping terrain, bridges, and rocks appear on your path. Do these moves carefully so you don't trip.*

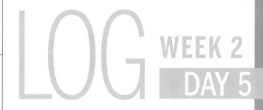

Date/Time of Day _____     **Miles Walked/Step Count** _____

**Program** _____     **Minutes Walked** _____

## A-B-C Daily Plan

☐ **ACCELERATED** (☐ INTENSE ☐ BRISK ☐ STEADY)   **interval ratio** _____

**number of intervals** _____

☐ **BODY SHAPING duration** _____

☐ **CARDIO duration** _____

## Location or Route _____

_____

_____

## Notes _____

_____

_____

_____

_____

_____

_____

_____

_____

_____

_____

# DAY 6

## HEED THE MALL'S CALL

For a safe, comfortable workout, check out your local mall. Like walking outdoors, walking at the mall is free. And many open early just for walkers. If yours doesn't, choose off-peak times for your walks to avoid crowds.

"Where you walk makes a difference," says Richard S. Cimbalo, PhD, professor of psychology at Daemen College in Amherst, New York. "Something about the mall—possibly that it's a familiar and safe place—may help women get a better workout."

But that's not the only advantage to walking in a mall. Here are some of the other reasons why you may want to take your exercise indoors.

**You're too hot.** As the temperature and humidity rise, your heart has to work harder to deliver blood not only to the muscles you're using but also to your skin to keep it cool. When exercising outdoors isn't safe, take advantage of air-conditioned malls. (See page 54.)

**You're too cold.** Cold presents its own problems, which may be complicated by icy or snowy sidewalks. Often, it's safer to drive than it is to walk. So drive yourself to the mall and walk there.

**You're sneezing.** In most malls, the air is filtered as well as cool and dry. So if you have allergies, you won't be bothered by pollen or dust as you would outdoors.

**You like company.** A growing number of malls sponsor organized walking programs, which may include group walks, special incentives, and even speakers and health fairs. To find out whether your local mall has such a program, call or stop by the administrative office.

**You want security.** A mall offers a smooth, even walking surface that's well lit and well populated. You can feel safe there. That's one of the big reasons why mall walking is becoming so popular, even in areas where the climate is mild.

**You're short on cash.** Walking in a mall is a lot less expensive than joining a health club or buying a treadmill.

### TIP

Make a game out of mall-walking. Memorize the order of the stores. Learn what's hot and what's not by checking out window-front items in music and clothing stores. If you are walking with a group, organize a treasure hunt where one person scouts out storefront items that other walkers must try to spot, suggests Thomas Cabot, president of the National Organization of Mall Walkers in Hermann, Missouri.

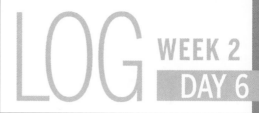

Date/Time of Day _____     Miles Walked/Step Count _____

Program _____     Minutes Walked _____

## A-B-C Daily Plan

☐ **ACCELERATED** (☐ INTENSE  ☐ BRISK  ☐ STEADY) **interval ratio** _____

**number of intervals** _____

☐ **BODY SHAPING duration** _____

☐ **CARDIO duration** _____

## Location or Route _____

_____

_____

## Notes _____

_____

_____

_____

_____

_____

_____

_____

_____

_____

_____

# DAY 7

## TAKE A GIANT STEP TOWARD SLIMNESS

Congratulations! You're halfway through your 4-week walking plan. By now there's a good chance that the results are starting to show on the scale and in the way that your clothes fit.

To maximize your efforts, adopt a "bottoms up" approach to life. That means you're always eager to get up and go, whether it's to walk down the hall to talk to a colleague instead of e-mailing her or to stand up and stretch while you're on the phone. The less you sit and the more you move, the more fit and healthy you'll be. Here are some easy ways to get more activity into your days.

**Don't park out front.** When Donna J. Kinoshita, 48, of Lafayette, Colorado, kept forgetting to walk, she finally decided to park her car a few blocks away from home. That way she had to walk. As she got in better shape, the car got farther and farther away from home, until finally she got rid of it and opted to walk everywhere. That was June of 1992. Kinoshita is fortunate enough to live in a town where many grocery stores, restaurants, and businesses are within walking distance. Also, if necessary, she can opt for public transportation. When Kinoshita is running late, she takes the bus. "I haven't had a car since 1992 and I love it," she says.

**Take commercial breaks.** There's about 10 minutes of commercials for every hour of television programming. So if you find yourself glued to Seinfeld reruns when you should be out walking, at least make a habit of doing circles around your coffee table during the commercials, says Peggy Norwood, an exercise physiologist, president of Avalon Fitness, and former fitness director of the Duke University Diet and Fitness Center, both in Durham, North Carolina.

**Do errands on foot.** One rule Norwood asks women to follow is the convenience-store rule. Find a convenience store that's within walking distance. Then when you need one item—say, you ran out of milk—don't drive. If you don't have a convenience store nearby, look for another destination that you often visit, such as a park, your hair salon, a school, or a friend's house. And use the bathroom and water fountain that's farthest away, preferably on another floor—take the stairs. If you have to take the car, get out of it as often as possible. Skip drive-thrus at banks and restaurants. Instead, park your car and go inside. And walk inside to pay for gas.

Get up from your desk. If you have a desk job, set a timer to alert you hourly. When it goes off, get up and take a walk, or simply stretch for a minute or two.

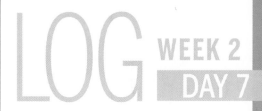

**Date/Time of Day** _____ **Miles Walked/Step Count** _____

**Program** _____ **Minutes Walked** _____

## A-B-C Daily Plan

☐ **ACCELERATED** (☐ INTENSE ☐ BRISK ☐ STEADY) **interval ratio** _____

**number of intervals** _____

☐ **BODY SHAPING duration** _____

☐ **CARDIO duration** _____

## Location or Route _____

_____

_____

## Notes _____

_____

_____

_____

_____

_____

T
I
P

*Plan now on how you're going to celebrate finishing your fourth week of walking. Maybe a massage, a new pair of shoes, or a night on the town with your partner or girlfriends? Choose something that you can look forward to, something that will inspire you for the next 2 weeks.*

# CHAPTER 7

# Week 3

**Weight** _____

**Pounds Lost** _____

# DAY 1

## REV UP TO DROP SIZES

In April 2002, Suzanne McCoy of Howell, New Jersey, quit smoking after 22 years and searched for a diet to lose weight. At 5 feet, 9 inches, and 262 pounds, she knew she had to make drastic changes. With a bad back and knees aching from arthritis, exercise didn't seem like an option. At first, she tried the Atkins Diet, under her doctor's supervision, and lost 60 pounds. But she just didn't like the food choices and felt it would not be something she could sustain for a lifetime. In addition, her cholesterol soared and her doctor put her on medications that gave her headaches and sapped her energy. She gained back 40 pounds. Next, she turned to Weight Watchers, finding the point system and variety of foods more compatible with her tastes and lifestyle, and dropped 28 pounds. That's when McCoy realized that she needed some kind of physical activity to maintain her weight loss and feel healthy and fit.

The minute she learned about the Presidential Sports Award Challenge (www. presidentialchallenge.org), she decided to go for it. The contest required that she walk every day.

To encourage her, McCoy's 12-year-old daughter, Becky, decided to join her. They walked together daily, keeping their own logs and enjoying each other's company and support. The reward? In addition to a certificate of achievement signed by President Bush, McCoy lost a total of 58 pounds, her cholesterol dropped into a healthy range, plus she felt energized and excited. "And the time to bond with my daughter was really satisfying," she says.

McCoy went on to earn additional awards and has completed five 10-mile walks and one 15-mile trek.

**Date/Time of Day** _____    **Miles Walked/Step Count** _____

**Program** _____    **Minutes Walked** _____

## A-B-C Daily Plan

☐ **ACCELERATED** (☐ INTENSE  ☐ BRISK  ☐ STEADY)  **interval ratio** _____

                                                    **number of intervals** _____

☐ **BODY SHAPING duration** _____

☐ **CARDIO duration** _____

## Location or Route _____

_____

_____

## Notes _____

_____

_____

_____

_____    

_____    

_____    

_____    **T I P**  *To boost the odds of fitting in your walks, do the same things at the same time every day. That includes going to bed, waking up, eating your meals, and taking your walk. It isn't always practical, but even doing it several times a week can help make walking a habit.*

_____    

_____

# DAY 2

## DON'T LET FEAR THWART YOUR WORKOUTS

Poorly lit streets, a dearth of sidewalks, and a lack of reachable destinations, such as parks and open spaces, can eat away at one's resolution to go out. And a new study from Ohio State University found that perceived neighborhood danger was the biggest reason women stay indoors.

To some aspiring walkers, such hurdles may loom larger than life. To our experts, they are mere bumps in the road. Here's how, with a little creativity and walking ingenuity, you can beat the obstacles standing between you and a daily walk.

### TAKE PRECAUTIONS

**Scope it out.** Try driving your planned route looking for danger zones. Look for unlit streets or corners where people loiter. Just be sure to canvass the area at the time of day you plan to be out walking. If you're still unsure about a route's safety, take a friend on your maiden voyage.

**Pack some heat.** Keep a can of pepper spray handy, says Liz Neporent, *Prevention* contributing editor and author of *Fitness Walking for Dummies*. Its punch comes from chile pepper oil. The spray is most effective when the target is within 10 feet. A 1-second blast to the face is enough to deter a dog—or anyone else, for that matter—for up to 45 minutes, which gives you plenty of time to get to safety. (And the pooch—or person—won't suffer any permanent damage.) You can buy pepper spray especially for walkers at www.pepper-spray-store.com.

**Outnumber 'em.** Dogs and bad guys are less likely to go after a group, says Neal Rawls, a security expert and author of *Be Alert, Be Aware, Have a Plan*. Try finding a walking group—or start your own.

### STAND OUT

Heading out for a walk is not the time to worry about whether you look too colorful or bright. Your clothing needs to be functional, even if this means you'll be wearing colors you usually wouldn't choose. There are plenty of options—just make sure you use them. Most pedestrian deaths happen at night, and research shows that walkers seriously overestimate how visible they are to drivers.

**Brighten up.** During the day, orange, red, and yellow are the colors most likely to attract a driver's attention. Before sunrise or after sunset, choose clothing made with reflective materials such as Illuminite, a high-tech light-reflective fabric that reflects the wearer's silhouette (www.illuminite.com). For a faster, cheaper fix, Neporent recommends buying reflective tape at a hardware store and sticking lots of it on a sweatshirt or jacket you reserve just for walking at sunrise or after sunset.

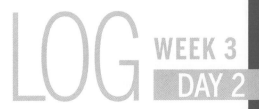

**Date/Time of Day** _____

**Program** _____

**Miles Walked/Step Count** _____

**Minutes Walked** _____

## A-B-C Daily Plan

☐ **ACCELERATED** (☐ INTENSE ☐ BRISK ☐ STEADY) **interval ratio** _____

**number of intervals** _____

☐ **BODY SHAPING duration** _____

☐ **CARDIO duration** _____

## Location or Route _____

_____

_____

## Notes _____

_____

_____

_____

_____

_____

_____

_____

_____

_____

**TIP**

*Avoid rush hour. Commuting hours are bad, day or night. Because many suburban and rural areas lack sidewalks, choosing light-traffic times is key. If you have to walk at high-traffic times, avoid busy streets that lack sidewalks and intersections without signals or crosswalks.*

# DAY 3

## MAKE YOUR WALKS MORE RELAXING

Research has linked stress to a host of physical ills, from back pain and stomach upset to high blood pressure and heart disease. But by participating in a regular walking program, you can offset the long-term health implications of stress.

Of course, when you're under pressure, whatever its source, going for a walk may be the last thing on your mind. You're not the only one who feels that way. When researchers tracked the exercise habits of 82 women for 8 weeks, they found that the women worked out less often during weeks that were filled with stressful events. At those times, exercise was "just one more thing to do."

When walking starts to feel like a stress-producer instead of a stress-reducer, try these workout adjustments to help you feel more relaxed and keep the pounds coming off.

**Adopt the right attitude.** Tell yourself that taking a walk will help you accomplish more on your "to-do" list. Exercise makes you feel better and think more clearly, so you become more productive.

**Aim for the morning.** Walking first thing in the morning, before anyone else is out and about, gives you an opportunity to focus on yourself, says Suki Munsell, PhD, director of the Dynamic Health and Fitness Institute in Corte Madera, California. "When my day looks hectic, with lots of decisions ahead, an early-morning walk brings answers and clarity," she notes.

**Seek out new scenery.** Choose a walking route that takes you down quiet streets or through a beautiful park. The more appealing your surroundings, the calmer you'll feel. Walking on busy streets, in unsafe neighborhoods, or after dark only adds to your stress.

**Slow your pace.** Pushing yourself to go faster or farther can add to your stress. During tense times, keep your walks leisurely.

**Focus on your breathing.** Taking deep breaths in time to your steps can make your walk more relaxing. Inhale as you take four to six steps and then exhale for four to six steps.

**Opt for a 10-minute trot.** At work, pass up the break-time doughnut and coffee and go for a walk instead. Research has shown that walking briskly can give you a bigger energy boost than eating a sugary snack. If you're able to go outside, the fresh air and sunshine can clear out those mental cobwebs and brighten your mood. If you can't get out, cruise the hallways of your workplace or climb a flight of stairs. You'll arrive back in your work area refreshed and ready to concentrate.

**Walk and talk.** Need to tackle a controversial issue with your spouse? Hesitant about discussing a sensitive topic with your daughter? Nervous about a meeting with a coworker? Take the conversation on the road. Walking will put both of you at ease because it relieves tension and anxiety—and you avoid direct eye contact. It may also stimulate new creative ideas for addressing the issues.

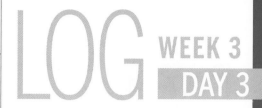

Date/Time of Day _____     Miles Walked/Step Count _____

Program _____     Minutes Walked _____

## A-B-C Daily Plan

☐ **ACCELERATED** ( ☐ INTENSE  ☐ BRISK  ☐ STEADY )  **interval ratio** _____

**number of intervals** _____

☐ **BODY SHAPING duration** _____

☐ **CARDIO duration** _____

## Location or Route _____

_____

_____

## Notes _____

_____

_____

_____

_____

_____

_____

_____

_____

**TIP**

*Walk away from a dilemma. When you're faced with a knotty problem that's left you feeling knotted up, think less and move more. Take a 10-minute leisurely stroll and let your mind wander. By the time you return to face the problem at hand, the answer that you were racking your brain for may seem obvious, and you've racked up some extra minutes on your walking plan.*

# DAY 4

## STAY INJURY FREE

We all know walking is the safest, easiest form of exercise there is, so why should you bother reading this? Because left ignored, an innocent niggle can easily become a chronic problem. In fact, nearly 250,000 hoofers a year are hobbled thanks to walking-induced pain or a nagging old wound that walking has aggravated.

Here's advice on avoiding and treating a common walking woe, plantar fasciitis. (For advice on other common walking injuries, see pages 92–94.)

Tenderness or pain on your heel or the bottom of your foot is a symptom of this problem. It's most severe in the morning or after sitting for a long time and decreases with activity.

The pain occurs when the fascia (a band of fibrous connective tissue on the bottom of the foot) becomes inflamed, often because of excessive pronation (rolling in of the foot and ankle) and poor-fitting shoes. It may also be caused by muscle imbalance, bone deformity, obesity, injury, and tightness in the calf muscle. If left untreated, the problem can cause a buildup of calcium, creating a painful, bony growth around the heel known as a heel spur.

At the first sign of

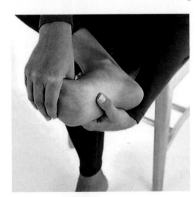

stiffness in the bottom of your foot, loosen up the tissue by performing this stretch regularly: Sit with the ankle of the injured foot across the opposite thigh. Pull the toes toward the shin until you feel a stretch in the arch. (See photo below.) Run your opposite hand along the sole of the foot; you should feel a taut band of tissue down the center. Do 10 stretches, holding each one for 10 seconds.

Do the stretches before getting out of bed in the morning and twice more during the day.

To reduce pain, wear shoes at all times. Choose walking shoes that are not too flexible in the middle. "They should be bendable at the ball but provide stiffness and support at the arch," says Melinda Reiner, DPM, vice president of the American Association for Woman Podiatrists. Using off-the-shelf orthotic inserts (Dr. Scholl's or Spenco, for example) or a custom-made pair can absorb some of the impact of walking, especially on hard surfaces.

Until you can walk pain free, stick to flat, stable, giving paths (such as a level dirt road), and avoid concrete, sand, or uneven ground that might cause too much flexing at the arch.

If pain persists, see your doctor.

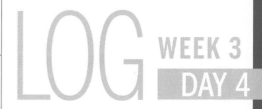

**Date/Time of Day** _____    **Miles Walked/Step Count** _____

**Program** _____    **Minutes Walked** _____

## A-B-C Daily Plan

☐ **ACCELERATED** (☐ INTENSE ☐ BRISK ☐ STEADY) **interval ratio** _____

**number of intervals** _____

☐ **BODY SHAPING duration** _____

☐ **CARDIO duration** _____

## Location or Route _____

_____

_____

## Notes _____

_____

_____    
_____    
_____    
_____    
_____    
_____    
_____

### TIP

*If you have cramping and burning in your calf muscles, try slowing your pace. If you're still in pain, stand facing the nearest wall or tree, then lean forward, putting your palms against the wall or tree and keeping your heels flat on the ground. Or sit on a bench with your legs straight out in front of you and flex your feet toward you. Still in pain? Hobble home and apply ice for 15 minutes. Be sure to wrap the ice in a towel to protect your skin from the cold.*

# DAY 5

## FROM 0 TO 60

Your body undergoes calorie-burning fluctuations and other changes every minute that you exercise. Here's what happens.

### MINUTES 1 TO 5

Your first few steps trigger the release of energy-producing chemicals in your cells to fuel your walk. Your heart rate revs from about 70 to 100 beats per minute (bpm), boosting blood flow and warming muscles. Any stiffness subsides as joints release lubricating fluid to help you move more easily. As you get moving, your body burns 3 calories per minute, compared with only 1 per minute at rest. Your body needs more fuel and starts pulling from its carb and fat stores.

### MINUTES 6 TO 10

Heartbeat increases from 100 to about 140 bpm, and you're burning up to 5 calories a minute as you pick up the pace. A slight rise in blood pressure is countered by the release of chemicals that expand blood vessels, bringing more blood and oxygen to working muscles.

### MINUTES 11 TO 20

Your body temperature keeps rising, and you start to perspire as blood vessels near the skin expand to release heat. As your walk becomes brisker, you'll be burning up to 9 calories a minute and breathing harder. Hormones such as epinephrine and glucagon rise to release fuel to the muscles.

### MINUTES 21 TO 45

Feeling invigorated, you start to relax as your body releases tension, thanks in part to a dose of feel-good chemicals such as endorphins in your brain. As more fat is burned, insulin (which helps store fat) drops—excellent news for anyone battling excess weight or diabetes.

### MINUTES 46 TO 60

Your muscles may feel fatigued as carb stores are reduced. As you cool down, your heart rate decreases and your breathing slows. You'll be burning fewer calories, but more than you were before you started. Your calorie burn will remain elevated for up to 1 hour.

## TIP

When it comes to giving you energy, carbs are the hands-down winner. The popularity of low-carb diets has given carbs a bad name, but there's no refuting the science. Your muscles are fueled by glycogen, which is a form of glucose—another name for sugar. Carbohydrates such as grains, fruits, and vegetables break down into sugar in your body, giving you nearly instant pep. But it's a short burst: Ultimately, your blood sugar will drop, which can make you feel fatigued. For staying power, combine your carbs with protein, which keeps your blood sugar on an even keel—and you moving— longer.

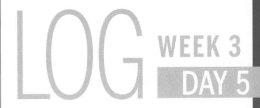

Date/Time of Day _____     Miles Walked/Step Count _____

Program _____     Minutes Walked _____

## A-B-C Daily Plan

☐ **ACCELERATED** ( ☐ INTENSE  ☐ BRISK  ☐ STEADY )  **interval ratio** _____

**number of intervals** _____

☐ **BODY SHAPING duration** _____

☐ **CARDIO duration** _____

## Location or Route _____

_____

_____

## Notes _____

_____

_____

_____

_____

_____

_____

_____

_____

_____

_____

_____

# DAY 6

## TRY THE ULTIMATE WALKING GEAR

Your fat cells and muscle tissue don't know whether you are walking outside or inside on a treadmill. So theoretically, walking on a treadmill should burn the same number of calories as walking on other surfaces.

In reality, however, most people burn more calories on a treadmill than walking elsewhere. Because treadmills force you to walk at an even clip, many walkers tend to walk slightly faster when indoors, thus burning more calories than when outside. And you keep your pace consistent. There's no stopping to smell the flowers, which means your calorie burn will stay revved up. Treadmills also offer other advantages.

- There are no sticks to trip over.
- There are no worries about walking too far away from home and not being able to make it back.
- Because of their cushioned rollers, some treadmills absorb about 40% of the jarring that you would get by walking on a road, making them joint-friendly.

- Because you use a treadmill indoors, you don't have to worry about the weather messing up your walking plans.
- And most important, many treadmills have a device to monitor your heart rate while you walk, so you can fine tune your workouts to an intensity that's right for you.
- Many manufacturers carry treadmills designed to absorb more shock. These models are often more expensive, but they're worth it if you're obese or have joint problems.

> **TIP**
>
> *If your treadmill has an incline function, use it to add oomph to your workout in short bursts—anywhere from 30 seconds to 3 minutes. When walking becomes laborious or you start losing good form, return to a flat position. Or you can slow your pace to adjust to the incline, just as you do when you're walking outdoors.*

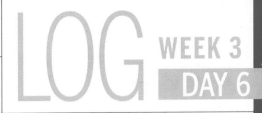

Date/Time of Day _____     **Miles Walked/Step Count** _____

Program _____     **Minutes Walked** _____

## A-B-C Daily Plan

☐ **ACCELERATED** (☐ INTENSE  ☐ BRISK  ☐ STEADY)  **interval ratio** _____

**number of intervals** _____

☐ **BODY SHAPING duration** _____

☐ **CARDIO duration** _____

## Location or Route _____

_____

_____

## Notes _____

_____

_____

_____

_____

_____

_____

_____

_____

_____

_____

# DAY 7

## LOOK 5 POUNDS SLIMMER

Virtually everything we do in modern life—from Internet surfing and desk work to driving and eating—rounds our bodies forward. And almost nothing we do reverses this curve, arching us back. As a result, poor posture is common and may contribute to a variety of ailments, from headaches to back spasms. And it can make you look and feel older and heavier than you really are.

Have you ever noticed that people who carry themselves with good alignment appear confident and graceful, while those whose posture reflects a physical slump often seem to be in a mental slump as well? Since our bodies and minds are linked, our posture mirrors our emotional state: When we're depressed, our bodies reflect this collapse. When we're happy, we look—and feel—like we're walking on air.

Stressful emotions can exert a subtle but damaging effect on posture. When we're chronically tense, certain muscles— often in the shoulders, back, and neck— are in a constant state of contraction, pulling the spine out of alignment and creating more stress. Learning to stand and sit with good posture can help muscles relax, which, in turn, can help the mind relax. Learning to lift your head and open your chest can lift your spirits as well. And it makes you look about 5 pounds thinner instantly.

Here's a simple posture exercise that you can do anywhere, anytime, standing or sitting, to open up the chest area and prevent rounded shoulders. Try it: Keeping your shoulders down, squeeze your shoulder blades together. Hold for about 10 seconds and repeat as often as possible. It may help you to imagine that you're using your shoulder blades to crack a walnut placed between them. Or pretend that you have a pencil balanced along your spine and squeeze your shoulder blades together to hold the pencil in place.

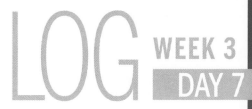

Date/Time of Day _____    **Miles Walked/Step Count** _____

Program _____    **Minutes Walked** _____

## A-B-C Daily Plan

☐ **ACCELERATED** (☐ INTENSE ☐ BRISK ☐ STEADY) **interval ratio** _____

                                             **number of intervals** _____

☐ **BODY SHAPING duration** _____

☐ **CARDIO duration** _____

## Location or Route _____

_____

_____

## Notes _____

_____

**TIP**

*Breathing exercises aren't just for yoga class. Concentrate on breathing in through your nose and out through your mouth for at least the first few minutes of each walk. Focus on drawing air into your belly first, before letting the air expand into your rib cage and chest. Deep, full breaths help relieve stress and energize your walk and your day.*

# CHAPTER 8

# Week 4

Weight _____

Pounds Lost _____

# DAY 1

## STAY FRIENDS WITH ROVER

If there are dogs in your neighborhood—even if you think they're harmless—it's a good idea to be prepared to protect yourself from an attack.

Every year, more than four million Americans are bitten by dogs. These bites and attacks can occur anytime, anywhere. Even dogs that seem friendly around their owners can become aggressive when they're protecting their turf from strangers. If you can take another route, do so. Or call local authorities—either your town's animal-control officer or the police—to find out the provisions of municipal leash laws and to report any violations.

If you must walk by a property with potentially dangerous dogs, be sure to carry something for protection. Tie a sweatshirt around your waist, wear a fanny pack, carry an umbrella or a walking stick—anything that you can put between yourself and a dog, in case one tries to bite you. The dog won't care if he gets you or the object in your hand. As he bites down on the object, keep tension on it and back yourself to a place of safety, like inside a car or behind a fence. Then let go and wait for him to leave.

Never stare down a dog. Instead, stand still and try to stay calm. Say, "No!" in a deep, firm voice. If the dog stops in his tracks, yell, "Go home!"

"Most dogs give warnings that you need to respect," says Randy Lockwood, PhD, of The Humane Society of the United States. Heed these danger signs of approaching dogs looking for a fight:

- Hard, intense stares
- Making a head-on approach to you
- Raised lip or snarl
- Tense body, tail held high and stiff, and standing forward on front toes

The best offense is still a good defense. Counter these postures by avoiding direct eye contact, moving slowly away in a diagonal direction (far from the aggressive dog's turf, such as his yard), offering treats tossed at a safe distance, and speaking in a calm, confident tone.

If a dog knocks you down, curl into a tight ball and protect your head and neck with your hands. Wait for the animal to leave, then slowly move to safety. Running will only attract the dog's attention. Report any attack to your local animal-control office immediately. Even if the dog bit your fanny pack and didn't harm you, he's dangerous, and his owner should be notified.

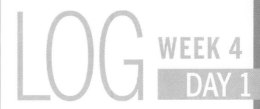

Date/Time of Day _____    **Miles Walked/Step Count** _____

Program _____    **Minutes Walked** _____

## A-B-C Daily Plan

☐ **ACCELERATED** (☐INTENSE ☐BRISK ☐STEADY) **interval ratio** _____

**number of intervals** _____

☐ **BODY SHAPING duration** _____

☐ **CARDIO duration** _____

## Location or Route _____

_____

_____

## Notes _____

_____

_____

_____

_____

_____

_____

_____

_____

_____

**T I P**

*If you just want a four-legged walking partner, not a full-time companion, ask friends and neighbors to "borrow" their dogs. Or contact your local animal shelter—often they're in need of volunteer dog walkers.*

*Many folks donate an hour after work or during lunch to get fresh air with Rover. For more information about volunteering, contact your local humane organization or SPCA.*

# DAY 2

## FAMILY MOTIVATES WALKER

Jerlynn Torres had always been overweight. "No one in my family ever exercised," says the native of Riverside, California, who recalls eating candy bars for breakfast and nachos for lunch as a kid. At 18, when her daughter, Alicia, was born, the 5-foot-4-inch Torres weighed 200 pounds; 4 months later, she was up to 224. She'd tried fad diets and diet pills but never got her weight below 200.

Then, 4 years ago, Alicia, just 5, came home in tears. The neighborhood kids, she explained between sobs, told her she was fat. It was the proverbial "aha!" moment for Torres, who realized her daughter, like so many American children, was headed for health problems. That afternoon, Torres shut off the TV and started taking Alicia for walks around their house after work. Alicia was so unaccustomed to exercise, Torres says, "the first time she broke a sweat, she didn't know what was happening. She said, 'Mommy, my hair is crying!'"

Torres is an administrator at Star Trac, a firm that makes fitness equipment. Though the company had encouraged staff members to exercise at work, she'd never taken them up on the offer. But after Alicia's run-in with the neighborhood kids, Torres started walking on the treadmill at the gym during her break. Her poor eating habits didn't change much, but she lost 30 pounds in a year. Exercise helped Alicia slim down too.

Not soon after losing the 30 pounds, Torres got pregnant with her son, Mylo, and gained all that weight back. By the time her maternity leave ended, Star Trac had hired a nutritionist to lead seminars on eating healthfully. Torres enrolled in the classes.

In the 3 years since, Torres has lost 40 pounds. Now at 157, she hopes to lose 20 more. These days, she exercises 90 minutes a shot, five times a week— walking solo or with the family, running, or taking a spinning class at work. Walking remains her favorite way to relax "When I'm running, all I can think about is running," she says, "but when I'm walking, my mind can drift. It puts things in perspective."

## TIP

For easy morning workouts, prepare before you go to bed.
- If you use a treadmill, make sure it's unfolded (if you keep it folded).
- Set out your workout clothes and shoes.
- Have your favorite CD ready to play.
- Fill your water bottle.
- Preset your coffeemaker for a postwalk treat.

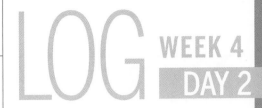
Date/Time of Day _____     **Miles Walked/Step Count** _____

**Program** _____     **Minutes Walked** _____

## A-B-C Daily Plan

☐ **ACCELERATED** (☐ INTENSE  ☐ BRISK  ☐ STEADY)  **interval ratio** _____

**number of intervals** _____

☐ **BODY SHAPING duration** _____

☐ **CARDIO duration** _____

## Location or Route _____

_____

_____

## Notes _____

_____

_____

_____

_____

_____

_____

_____

_____

_____

# DAY 3

## BEAT BOREDOM

What are you doing today? Are you doing interval training, body shaping, or a cardio workout? Whatever is on the agenda, do you know the moves—or the route around the neighborhood—so well that your workouts are getting tedious? And an outdoor track, while keeping you safe from dogs and cars, lacks variety.

Here are some ideas to mix things up.

**Seek out happy trails.** A change of scenery may be just what you need. Women who live near trails or walking paths are 38% more active than those who don't. None in your neighborhood? Check out local hiking trails, Rails-to-Trails paths, or canal towpaths. The uneven terrain will give your body a new kind of workout, and the beautiful surroundings will give your mind a much-needed break. Or search out botanical gardens, fairgrounds, zoos, college campuses, orchards, and reservoirs in your area; then hoof it to one of these destinations before the end of the month.

**Jot down your motives.** Come up with five, and store them in a jar or decorative box. The next time you don't feel like exercising, pick one. Reading reminders such as "Fit into dress for daughter's wedding," "Lower cholesterol," or "Sign up for 5-K" may be just the jump start you need to get out the door.

**Move to the beat.** Listening to up-tempo music can keep you strutting faster. "Music distracts you from thinking about how hard you're working. And it boosts your mood, making you more likely to keep going," says Robert T. Herdegen, PhD, Elliott Professor of psychology at Hampden-Sydney College in Virginia.

When walking on the treadmill became tedious for Kathy O'Connor, 54, of Peekskill, New York, she bought a music player that fits into a carrying case attached to her belt. Then she popped in some tunes she hadn't listened to in a while and was amazed at the difference. "You really can get lost in the music," says O'Connor. She suggests trying books on tape as well.

**Go for a moonwalk.** Don reflective clothing, grab your partner and a flashlight, and head out for a midnight parade. Night noises and a starry sky will renew an old routine, and working out with someone is hands down more fun than traipsing around town alone.

**Explore new neighborhoods.** Drive to a nearby town that you've never walked around. Park your car and start exploring. Window-shop as you walk along the main street. Venture down side streets and check out the architecture, landscaping, and unique decorations—steal a few ideas for your home.

**Make it a date.** Invite a friend, your spouse, a parent, or one of your children to walk with you. Take advantage of this opportunity for a little one-on-one time to catch up, without all the distractions of home or the calories of meeting for lunch or dinner. You may even be so busy talking that you'll end up walking longer than you had planned!

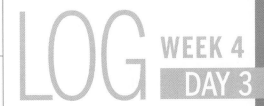

# LOG

**Date/Time of Day** _____    **Miles Walked/Step Count** _____

**Program** _____    **Minutes Walked** _____

## A-B-C Daily Plan

☐ **ACCELERATED** (☐ INTENSE ☐ BRISK ☐ STEADY) **interval ratio** _____

**number of intervals** _____

☐ **BODY SHAPING duration** _____

☐ **CARDIO duration** _____

## Location or Route _____

_____

_____

## Notes _____

_____

_____

_____

_____

_____

_____

_____

_____

T
I
P

*Good walking form makes quickening your pace a snap, says walking expert Mark Fenton, author of* The Complete Guide to Walking for Health, Fitness, and Weight Loss. *Bend your elbows. You wouldn't run with straight arms; don't fitness walk with them, either. Pump your arms so your fists swing in an arc from your waistband to chest height. Spring off your toes. Push off as though you were trying to show someone behind you the sole of your shoe with every step.*

# DAY 4

## REMEMBER WHY YOU STARTED

A little over 2 weeks ago, you embarked on a new adventure, one aimed at slimming down, getting toned, and improving your health. By now you know that walking is a giant step toward your goals. As you approach the finish line, you might want to remind yourself why you started in the first place.

Easy, convenient, low-cost, and injury free, walking is the one exercise that women can stick with.

Just ask Roseanne Welsh Strull. The day she decided to go for her first walk, she got her 272-pound frame off her living-room chair, went to the front door, opened it, stepped onto her driveway, ambled down to her mailbox, turned around, ambled back up the driveway, entered the house, closed the door, and returned to her living-room chair. "There," she told herself. "I did it. Now all I have to do is do it again tomorrow."

Today, Strull weighs 135 pounds. Walking to the mailbox poses no struggle. Neither does aerobics class, a bicycle ride, a round of badminton, or a night on the dance floor. In fact, Strull has been so successful at losing weight that—as a personal trainer and lifestyle counselor in Beaverton, Oregon, the author of *Thinner Winners*, and now many years at her goal—she teaches other women how to use exercise to do the same.

Though she has branched out since her early exercise days, Strull chose walking as her first exercise because it was the only aerobic activity that she knew how to do. And all she needed to get herself started was a good pair of shoes. Once she started, walking never let her down.

Strull started walking for the same reasons that so many other women choose it as their aerobic activity.

**Walking sticks.** Studies show that four out of five women who walk for exercise keep walking. In contrast, half of the women who try other types of exercise, like swimming, stair climbing, or running, call it quits during the first few months.

**Walking is gentle.** Many overweight women simply cannot do activities such as jogging or aerobic dance because their joints cannot handle the pounding. But most overweight women can walk, says William Joel Wilkinson, MD, medical director of the division of epidemiology and clinical applications at the Cooper Institute for Aerobics Research in Dallas.

**Walking is an easy fit.** Walking is one of the easiest activities to fit into a busy day, says John M. Jakicic, PhD, research assistant professor in psychiatry at the University of Pittsburgh. When you split it up into short increments, walking can be squeezed into your day before breakfast or during lunch and coffee breaks at work. You don't have to take the time to change clothes or shower. And you can do it anytime, anywhere. It's as easy as circling your backyard—or your living-room coffee table.

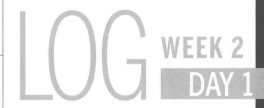

Date/Time of Day _____     Miles Walked/Step Count _____

Program _____     Minutes Walked _____

## A-B-C Daily Plan

☐ **ACCELERATED** (☐ INTENSE  ☐ BRISK  ☐ STEADY)  **interval ratio** _____

**number of intervals** _____

☐ **BODY SHAPING duration** _____

☐ **CARDIO duration** _____

## Location or Route _____

_____

_____

## Notes _____

_____

_____

_____

_____

_____

_____

_____

_____

_____

**TIP**

*Minute per minute, walking at a brisk pace burns about the same number of calories as low-impact aerobics.*

# DAY 5

## TAKE CARE OF YOUR FEET

By now, you've been pounding a lot of pavement, and your feet deserve a break. If you're like most people, you probably just walk all over them. But taking them for granted for too long can have painful consequences: 75% of Americans get foot pain at some point, and women's feet are four times more likely to hurt. But the good news is that many of these problems are avoidable. Here's how to keep your feet happy.

• Wear appropriate shoes for the activity you are performing: well-cushioned shoes for long periods of standing and activity-specific shoes for exercise.

• Stick with heels no higher than 3/4". High heels contribute to knee and back problems, falls, and an awkward, unnatural gait. In time, they may cause enough changes in your feet to impair proper function.

• Avoid tight socks or nylons that squeeze your toes or bunch under your feet.

• Massage your feet at least once a week. Put a small, sturdy glass bottle or a golf ball on the floor and roll it under your foot, bearing down with a little pressure. (Chill the bottle or ball for added relief.) Or splurge on a professional foot massage occasionally.

• Give your toes a good stretch at the end of the day by interlacing the fingers of your right hand between the toes of your left foot. Hold for a minute or so, then switch feet.

**TIP**

*Add a racewalking hip swivel to increase speed, trim your waistline, and burn more calories: Walk slowly, crossing your feet slightly in front of you so one hip rotates forward while the other goes back. (Think runway models, but don't exaggerate your movements as much.) Once you get the feel, pick up the pace and try it without crossing your feet.*

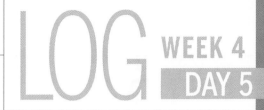

**Date/Time of Day** _____    **Miles Walked/Step Count** _____

**Program** _____    **Minutes Walked** _____

## A-B-C Daily Plan

☐ **ACCELERATED** (☐ INTENSE ☐ BRISK ☐ STEADY) **interval ratio** _____

**number of intervals** _____

☐ **BODY SHAPING duration** _____

☐ **CARDIO duration** _____

## Location or Route _____

_____

_____

## Notes _____

_____

_____

_____

_____

_____

_____

_____

_____

_____

_____

# DAY 6

## CALORIES GO, FAST OR SLOW

The chart at right compares the number of calories burned by an average 150-pound person while walking at various speeds. As you can see, the faster you go, the more calories you use per minute. But if you figure out the number of calories burned per mile, there's not that much difference between walking slow and walking fast.

For example, a 20-minute-per-mile pace burns 3.7 calories per minute, or 74 calories per mile (20 x 3.7 = 74). By comparison, a 12-minute-per-mile pace burns 9.1 calories per minute, or 109 calories per mile (12 x 9.1 = 109.2). That's just 35 calories more—and you can easily make up for that by walking an extra 1/2 mile at the slower pace.

So if you're walking to lose weight, remember that you don't need to push yourself at top speed. Going slower but farther—long, slow distance—can produce the same results.

## CALORIE BURN

| Speed (MPH) | Minutes per Mile | Calories Burned per Minute |
|---|---|---|
| 2.0 | 30.0 | 2.8 |
| 2.5 | 24.0 | 3.4 |
| 3.0 | 20.0 | 3.7 |
| 3.5 | 17.1 | 4.3 |
| 4.0 | 15.0 | 5.7 |
| 4.5 | 13.2 | 7.1 |
| 5.0 | 12.0 | 9.1 |

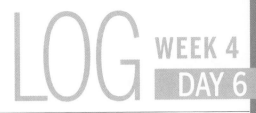

**Date/Time of Day** _____

**Miles Walked/Step Count** _____

**Program** _____

**Minutes Walked** _____

## A-B-C Daily Plan

☐ **ACCELERATED** (☐ INTENSE ☐ BRISK ☐ STEADY) **interval ratio** _____

**number of intervals** _____

☐ **BODY SHAPING duration** _____

☐ **CARDIO duration** _____

## Location or Route _____

_____

_____

## Notes _____

_____

_____

_____

_____

_____

_____

_____

_____

_____

**TIP**

*If you really want to walk, you'll find the time. It's not really any different than finding time to eat, for instance. Think about it: Don't you always have time for that? You can do the same with walking—consider it a necessity, not an optional activity.*

# DAY 7

## DON'T STOP NOW!

If you've walked most every day this month, you're well on your way to making walking for weight loss a habit. To keep up your motivation, pick a specific goal to strive for, such as walking a half or full marathon or taking a walking vacation in a beautiful, exciting locale. To find walker-friendly marathons, visit www.prevention.com/walking.

Walking vacations are great ways to visit interesting places you've read about—and get some exercise. Below is a list of walks that get top billing year after year in a contest held by the American Volkssport Association. For more information and directions for any of these walks, or to find great walking trails in other parts of the country go to www.ava.org or call (800) 830-WALK (9255).

**West Point, New York:** Starting at USMA Visitors Center on West Point Highway, the walk winds along the West Point Military Academy campus, takes you past historic monuments, and offers great views of the Hudson River. The trail ranked number one 2 years in a row.

**South Portland, Maine:** Starting at Hannaford's Supermarket on Cottage Road, the route winds along local sidewalks, pathways, and beaches, allowing you to see many of the area's famed lighthouses and offering a beautiful view of the capes.

**San Antonio, Texas:** Starting at El Tropicano Riverwalk Hotel on Lexington Avenue, this trail goes along the Riverwalk through the city's King William District, the Hemisfair Park, and the historic Alamo.

**Devils Tower, Wyoming:** The trail starts at Devils Tower Trading Post and takes you through and around Devils Tower, the first landmark in the United States to be declared a national monument.

**Guernsey, Wyoming:** Starting at Guernsey State Park on Highway 26, the walk runs along a section of the famous Oregon Trail, where ruts left behind by early settlers are still visible.

**Washington, DC:** Starting at Columbia Plaza Apartments on 23rd Street, this popular walk takes you along city streets and through historic monument sections. You'll get to see the Lincoln Memorial, the Washington Monument, the Capitol Building, the White House, and the Vietnam Memorial.

**Alexandria, Virginia:** The walk goes through the historic Old Town of Alexandria, on city sidewalks, and through parks along the Potomac River. The town dates back to the seventeenth and eighteenth centuries.

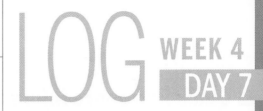

**Date/Time of Day** _____          **Miles Walked/Step Count** _____

**Program** _____          **Minutes Walked** _____

## A-B-C Daily Plan

☐ **ACCELERATED** (☐ INTENSE  ☐ BRISK  ☐ STEADY)  **interval ratio** _____

**number of intervals** _____

☐ **BODY SHAPING duration** _____

☐ **CARDIO duration** _____

## Location or Route _____

_____

_____

## Notes _____

_____

_____

_____

_____

_____

_____

_____

_____

**TIP**

*For a double dose of feel-good vibes, lend your feet to a cause. Training for and completing a charity walk with a large group is exhilarating; knowing you're ticking off a good deed in the process makes your success all the sweeter. And committing to an event will help ensure you keep up your walking program.*

# ■ Quick Reference Injury Guide

## ACHILLES TENDINITIS

**Symptom:** Pain at the back or sides of the heel without a bump, and in the lower calf. Pain can radiate into the ankle area and be sharp when walking.

**Causes:** The Achilles tendon, which connects the calf muscle to the heel, can be aggravated by walking too much, especially if you don't build up to it. The Achilles tendon can also be strained by repeatedly flexing the foot when walking up and down steep hills or uneven terrain.

**Treatment:** Rest, ice, anti-inflammatory medication for acute pain, and daily gentle stretching.

For mild cases, reduce your mileage—or substitute non–weight-bearing activities like weight training and cycling, so long as these don't aggravate the pain. Regular calf stretches will also minimize stress on the tendon, says Michael J. Mueller, PT, PhD, associate professor in physical therapy at the Washington University School of Medicine in St. Louis. In severe cases, stop walking and place cold packs on the injured area. When you return to walking, keep the foot in neutral position by sticking to flat surfaces.

## ANKLE SPRAIN

**Symptoms:** Most symptoms occur after you have twisted your ankle in a pretty obvious and painful way. You may have felt a "pop" at the time of the injury. You may experience swelling and bruising and feel pain when you put weight on the injured foot.

**Cause:** Stretching or tearing the ligaments on the outside of your ankle. Often occurs in people who have a high arch.

**Treatment:** Use the RICE method to help reduce swelling and pain in the first 48 hours: Rest your ankle by not walking on it; Ice it to keep the swelling down (20 minutes on, 40 minutes off cycle); Compress the area by lightly wrapping an Ace bandage around it; elevate it so your foot is higher than your waist. But don't use this injury as an excuse to avoid working out completely. "When doctors recommend RICE, they don't mean sitting in the La-Z-Boy for weeks," says sports medicine specialist Steven D. Stovitz, MD, of the University of Minnesota, who prefers the term *MICE*, swapping *motion* for *rest*. Increased blood circulation delivers more nutrients and removes more wastes from the injury site. The MICE secret: Avoid activities that aggravate the injured area; for example, trade walking for swimming. If the swelling and pain are severe or have not decreased after 48 hours, see a doctor or podiatrist to x-ray the area.

## BUNION

**Symptom:** Pain on the bony side of your big toe.

**Cause:** Bunions develop when the bones in the joint on the outside, lower end of the big or little toe become misaligned, forming a painful swelling that develops into a lump. While the condition is often genetic, walkers who have flat feet, low arches, or arthritis may be more prone to it.

**Treatment:** "Wear shoes that are wider—especially in the toe box," says Phillip Ward, DPM, a podiatrist in Pinehurst, North Carolina. If you don't want to shell out for new shoes, ask your shoe repair shop to stretch your old ones. Padding the bunion with over-the-counter bunion pads can also provide relief, and icing it for 20 minutes after walking will numb the area. Ultrasound or other physical therapy treatments may reduce bunions. Severe cases may require surgery to pare down the bone and realign the toe joint.

## BURSITIS

**Symptom:** Pain on the outside of your hips.

**Causes:** It's common for the fluid-filled sacs (bursa) that provide cushioning to the hip joints to become inflamed with repetitive stress. People with one leg slightly longer than the other are more prone to this condition. Too much walking without building up to it can also be a cause.

**Treatment:** Instead of walking, ride a stationary bike, swim, or do some other non–weight-bearing activity for a few weeks, says Frank Kelly, MD, an orthopedic surgeon in Macon, Georgia, and spokesperson for the American Academy of Orthopaedic Surgeons. He also suggests an anti-inflammatory medication uch as ibuprofen to reduce swelling in the tissue. When you begin walking again, don't just step back n where you left off. Start gradually by walking every ther day at first. Spend the first 5 minutes warming p by walking slowly, and do the last 5 minutes at a lower, cool-down pace," he says.

## FLAT FEET (LOW ARCH)

**Symptoms:** Pain after long periods of standing. Difficulty standing on the tiptoes of the affected foot. Your foot aches, particularly in the heel or arch area, nd you may have swelling along the inner side.

**Causes:** Heredity, diabetes, arthritis, or injury to muscles and tendons of the foot.

**Treatment:** Having flat feet is a serious matter. If ou're experiencing pain and think it's related to flat eet, see your podiatrist for a physical examination, gait analysis, and x-rays to determine if surgery or rthotics would be helpful.

## HAMMERTOE

**Symptoms:** One or more of your toes is permanently ent at the first joint. It may be painful to wear shoes, nd you may have corns on the top of these toes.

**Causes:** Tight shoes, high heels, and nylons that queeze the toes. Heredity and arthritis can also e factors.

**Treatment:** There are hammertoe pads available at rugstores that can help reduce pressure. Ice can ase acute pain. Wear a shoe that has lots of room the toe area, and avoid high-heeled shoes. These uggestions will provide relief, but you'll need to see podiatrist to discuss treatment options such as ping and padding the hammertoe, custom orthotic evices (supports or braces for problem joints r muscles), or surgical procedures to repair the ffected toe.

## HEEL SPUR

**Symptom:** Sharp pain on the bottom of your heel hen walking.

**Cause:** Often accompanies plantar fasciitis and is result of repeated tearing away of the membrane at is attached to the heel bone, resulting in the evelopment of a bony protrusion (spur).

**Treatment:** Properly fitted shoes can reduce ritation, but you should see a podiatrist for an x-ray

evaluation to assess the need for further treatment, surgery, or appropriate pain medication.

## HIGH ARCH

**Symptoms:** Rigid, bony foot that is hard to fit into shoes. You're prone to ankle sprains or twisted ankles and may experience generalized pain under the ball of the foot and in your heel area.

**Cause:** Heredity.

**Treatment:** Wear shoes that provide lots of cushioning and support. Avoid very rigid shoes.

## INGROWN TOENAIL

**Symptom:** Soreness or swelling on the sides of toes.

**Causes:** A tender tootsie can develop when the corners or sides of your toenails grow sideways rather than forward, putting pressure on surrounding soft tissues and even growing into the skin. You may be more prone to ingrown toenails if your shoes are too short or too tight, which causes repeated trauma to the toe as you walk, says Ward. If the excess pressure goes on too long, such as on a long hike or charity walk, the toenail may even fall off.

**Treatment:** Leave wiggle room in your shoes by going up a half or full size when you buy sneakers, since feet tend to swell during exercise. Use toenail clippers (not fingernail clippers or scissors) to cut straight across instead of rounding the corners. "People who overpronate when they walk can aggravate the big toes," says Ward, who suggests using inserts to reduce pronation. If you have diabetes or any circulatory disorder, have your ingrown toenails treated by a podiatrist (find one at www.apma.org).

## RUNNER'S KNEE

**Symptom:** Pain in the front of the kneecap.

**Cause:** Your kneecap may rub against your femur (the bone that connects your knee to your hip),

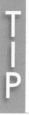

*This is a general guide intended to provide information about and treatment for common ailments. If pain persists or interferes with your daily activities, see your doctor.*

causing cartilage damage, inflammation, and tendinitis. Walkers with a misaligned kneecap, prior injury, weak or imbalanced thigh muscles, soft knee cartilage, or flat feet, or who simply do too much walking, may be prone to runner's knee. The pain usually appears when walking downhill, or doing knee bends, or during prolonged sitting.

**Treatment:** Shift to other exercise until the pain subsides, typically 8 to 12 weeks. Do some quad strengtheners two or three times a week to help align the kneecap and enhance support around the knee: Sit with back against a wall, right leg bent with foot flat on floor and left leg straight in front of you. Contract quads and lift left leg, keeping foot flexed. Repeat 12 times; work up to three sets per leg. While standing, place a looped band around both feet and sidestep 12 to 15 times to right, then back to left. When walking or hiking downhill, be sure to maintain good form by bending your knees before each step so that the thighs—not the knees—absorb the impact.

## SIDE STITCH

**Symptom:** A sudden, stabbing pain in your side while you're exercising.

**Cause:** A side stitch is a spasm of the diaphragm, the muscle that separates your chest and abdomen. This muscle is crying out for oxygen because your expanded lungs and contracted abdomen are blocking normal blood flow. This sounds serious, but it's not a big deal.

**Treatment:** At the first sign of a side stitch, stop walking. Using three fingers, massage the area where the pain is most severe until you feel relief. Do not hold your breath. As your breathing slows to its normal rate, the pain should subside. Then you can resume your walk. Like any muscle, your diaphragm cramps when it's not warmed up properly. So remember to warm up before you head out. Walking slowly should do the trick.

## STRAIN

**Symptom:** Pain without bruising in the ankle area. Not as severe as a sprain.

**Causes:** Usually due to excessive training, such as running or walking long distances without resting

enough, or wearing poor-quality shoes. Can lead to stress fractures.

**Treatment:** Use the RICE and MICE methods, described under "Ankle Sprain."

## STRESS FRACTURE

**Symptom:** Pinpoint pain in your foot or lower leg. If you feel tenderness or pain when you press with your fingers on a specific spot on your foot or lower leg, you may have a stress fracture—a tiny crack in a bone.

**Causes:** Such fractures, most common in the lower leg, tend to occur when the leg muscles become overloaded from repetitive stress and the bone absorbs the shock rather than the muscle. This can happen if you ignore a shin splint, for instance; the continued strain on muscles and tissues will eventually be shifted to the bone.

Walking is more apt to lead to a stress fracture if you're overweight or have low bone density, says Byron Russell, PhD, chair of the department of physical therapy at Eastern Washington University in Spokane. The National Osteoporosis Foundation recommends that those who experience frequent fractures get a bone density test. People with high arches or rigid flat feet may be more susceptible, and women are more vulnerable.

**Treatment:** Kick back and let the area heal for at least 6 to 8 weeks. "You need lots of rest to avoid loading the bones," says Sheila Dugan, MD, a physiatrist and assistant professor at Rush Medical College in Chicago. When you start up again, be sure to stop exercising before you feel any discomfort. "If you walk 1 mile and experience the onset of symptoms again, then start walking at one quarter of a mile and take several weeks to build up to the longer distance," says Russell. Replace worn walking shoes to ensure that you have adequate shock absorption. Also, to optimize bone health, do some lower-body strength training twice a week and eat calcium-rich foods like yogurt, cheese, and greens such as kale, or take a supplement. Women are advised to get 1,000 mg/day (or 1,200 mg/day for those 51 years and older).

*NOTE:* See page 27 for information on Morton's neuroma and page 70 for plantar fasciitis.

# Index

Note: <u>Underscored</u> page references indicate boxed text. **Bold** page references indicate photographs.